Second Opinion

Other books by Bruce Hilton

My Brother Is a Stranger
The Delta Ministry
Highly Irregular
Ethical Issues in Human Genetics (editor)
First, Do No Harm
Can Homophobia Be Cured?

Second Opinion

Reflecting

on Contemporary

Issues in Bioethics

Bruce Hilton

Abingdon Press / Nashville

Library of Congress Cataloging in Publication Data

Hilton, Bruce.
    Second opinion: reflecting on contemporary issues in bioethics / Bruce Hilton.
      p. cm.
    ISBN 0-687-07359-6 (alk. paper)
    1. Medical ethics. 2. Bioethics. I. Title

    R724 .H535 2001
    174'.2—dc21   2001018180

Study guide by John D. Schroeder

*To those who have filled out
an advance directive and thus saved
the doctors, nurses, and their own
distraught kin a peck of trouble*

Contents

Acknowledgments

For keeping my feet on the ground in hundreds of case discussions, hearty thanks to the Ethics Committees with whom I consult, and especially their wise and patient chairs, including Martin Janis, M.D., Khosrow Afsari, M.D., Peter Navolanic, M.D., Robert Herrick, M.D. and Howard Slyter, M.D.

For lending her eyes, judgment and experience throughout the process, from research to page proofs, boundless gratitude to the Reverend Virginia Y. Hilton, M.A., M.Div., R.N.

Most of these commentaries are adapted from my column, "Bioethics," nationally distributed the last fifteen years by Scripps Howard News Service. Scripps Howard's assistant managing editor, Walter Veazey, rescued the column from a watery grave after its original venue sank without a trace beneath the waves. Thanks, Walter!

Introduction

All I could see was the ceiling, rolling past overhead. Green like every other hospital ceiling.

I couldn't see who else was along on this slow cruise through the halls, but I could hear them talking quietly. Somebody was pushing the gurney; somebody else was opening doors for us. Another was acting as tour guide.

"Each room we go through is a little cooler," she said. "The operating room will be quite cool. That slows down your metabolism. Oh, and also helps prevent infection."

She was talking to me, but I had trouble believing it was me. This was the sort of thing that happened to other people, not to me.

We rolled to a stop. On the count of three, they lifted me to the cool metal operating table.

"Are you cold?" Somebody tucked a warmed blanket around my legs and hips.

Is this me? I thought.

Somebody connected a flat board to the left side of the table, at my shoulder, and fastened the outstretched left arm to it, palm up.

Nobody was barking orders, as in television. People moved quietly in and out of my vision. They do a thousand of these a year at this hospital, I reminded myself.

"Would you like a pillow? Might be a little more comfortable while we're getting ready."

I thought of the half-dozen columns in which I had criticized the thousands of unnecessary coronary bypass operations done in the United States each year.

"I'm going to use this wide belt to hold your legs in place," somebody said.

Somebody lifted my right arm and fastened it, outstretched, to another narrow board. Lying here, bound in place, I felt like the lead actor in a Good Friday pageant.

The man at my right leaned forward so I could see his eyes above the green mask.

"So," he said. "They tell us you're a bioethicist. What exactly does a bioethicist do?"

*   *   *

I was asleep before I could answer. But the question came back to me twenty-four hours later, along with a second question: What would Doc Devine have thought of all this?

Doc was the first physician I'd ever met. Measles, I think it was. Ma cranked the telephone on the wall with Doc's number (two longs and a short) and asked him to come over.

He didn't live far away. Nobody did in Ontario, Wisconsin (population 398, if you believe the sign at the edge of town).

Doc came over, looked at my rash, and told my folks to keep me in a dark room, to protect my eyes.

Then he gave my dad a bright red sign that said. "QUARANTINED" and asked him to tack it up on the front door. Nobody could visit us, and we couldn't leave the house for two weeks.

That was pretty much what a doctor could do in those days, make the patient comfortable, try to avoid additional harm, and try to keep disease from spreading to other families. Since a high percentage of the illness was contagious, he had to be both personal physician and public health officer.

He had no antibiotics; no doctor did. There were no transplants, no kidney machines, no intensive care units.

Within a few years, inoculation would do away with measles and mumps, and many of the other most common contagious diseases. On the other hand, the next generations of physicians would struggle with frustrating chronic diseases—many of them incurable. Ironically, these would grow in importance as modern medicine extended the average life expectancy. Longer lives meant more diseases of old age and longer suffering with chronic diseases that began in childhood.

The diseases changed, and so did the doctor-patient relationship. Doc's fellow physicians were shamans—priestly figures to whom the patient figuratively knelt in supplication. Much of their ability to heal depended on the patient's belief that it could happen. They rarely questioned the doctor's judgment.

If Doc could come back, he'd be astounded at how uppity we patients have become.

The civil rights movement told us we were equal, and the women's movement told us we were, nonetheless, unique individuals. When we took this new self-image to the doctor's office, something had to change.

And it did. Laypeople and physicians alike are learning that patients bring unique and valuable knowledge to any discussion with their doctors. They bring the one thing no medical school professor could have taught the doctor: their attitudes, wishes, and experiences—information essential for solving the complex moral questions.

Which brings us back to bioethics.

A bioethicist is someone trained to help patients or their surrogates look at all sides of a moral question, and then supports them in the decisions they make.

Bioethics is the study of the questions of right and wrong that arise in science and medicine. These questions are intriguing enough in their own right, but there's a practical reason that bioethicists are determined to help as many laypeople as possible learn how these decisions are made: because almost all of us will face questions like these someday in our own lives.

If my child is permanently unconscious, being kept alive only with a breathing machine, who has the right to turn off the machine—and for what reasons?

Your dying, unconscious father has asked, in advance, not to receive life support. But when everything but intravenous liquids and nutrients are withdrawn, he continues breathing. Would it be murder to cut off his water and food?

I hope this book helps satisfy your curiosity about such questions. I hope, too, that it helps you get ready to answer them when the patient is you, or somebody you care about.

Sacramento, California
November 13, 2000

Part One | Decisions

Is There Anything I Can Do?

What do you do when a friend is really sick? Long-term sick, maybe even terminal? Believe it or not, most other people don't know what to do, either. The practical suggestions in the list below come from several sources, especially the Center for Hospice and Palliative Care, Cheektowaga, N.Y.; the *British Medical Journal*; and *Coming Home*, by Deborah Duda.

Don't avoid the patient. Just be the friend you always have been. Illness can be a lonely time. If your friend slips away before that visit you keep postponing, the guilt hangs around a long time; believe me, I know.

Don't forget the family. They suffer too. If there are children, take them places. If adults in the family are giving the care, offer to come and stay with the patient while they get a break.

Don't avoid talk about the future. Hope is essential, even to those patients who know they won't be around for the coming year.

Have an open heart. Defined by Duda as "love without conditions and judgments. Not I love you if . . . Just 'I love you.' " The sick often are the subjects of blame. "You should have . . ." Forget it. A welcome side effect: We hear the patient much better when we have an open heart.

Water the flowers. Help with the cleaning or the yard; life goes on in the household. The best approach: Ask what you might do to help, and then follow through by doing it. Take the patient out for a pleasure trip. But know his or her limitations. Avoid something too strenuous or too long. You can't go wrong visiting a favorite view site. Ask for a shopping list. Then make a special delivery to the home.

Touch. There's no lonelier place than a severe illness, especially one that might be fatal. The Cheektowaga facility quotes a patient: "A simple squeeze of the hand tells me you still care." This can be especially important if the patient has cancer or HIV/AIDS. The latter isn't contagious in normal contact and cancer not at all, but studies show that prejudice is widespread. Anxious callers who keep their distance can do great emotional harm. Remember the open heart.

Be a chauffeur. The patient (or children or elderly parents) might need transportation to the hospital for a treatment, or to the doctor's office. Just as important, he or she may want to see an old friend. Ask where they'd like to go, and arrange to take them.

Remember that dying is okay. Pretending that death is not a possibility forces patients into a painful charade. Patients who are gravely ill know it. Pretending isolates them from their family and friends, and heightens the loneliness. Visitors who resist a patient's dying, or even urge the patient to hang on, and not "give up," are denying the realities. Worse, they heighten the patient's guilt. "The ultimate gift of love," to paraphrase Duda, "is letting someone die in their own way."

Ask. We like to assume we know how a patient feels. Even doctors, according to research done several years ago, believed they knew what kind of end-of-life treatment their patients wanted—but were wrong two-thirds of the time. Ask patients whether they want to be alone or with you. Ask whether they are "up" or "down," and accept the answer. Ask, "Is there anything I can do for you?"

Be creative. The Hospice Center suggests: bring a book of thoughts, taped music, a poster for the wall, cookies to share with family and friends. Be free to talk. Maybe the patient wants to talk. Ask, "Do you feel like talking about it?" Be free not to talk. Just being together quietly is good, too. Duda calls it "making space for what is happening."

He/she is still a person. Discuss all decisions about the patient with the patient. Do this even for the small things; it helps them keep a sense of dignity and worth. Encourage them to protect their decision-making rights with a Durable Power of Attorney for Health Care Decisions. But, if they resist, respect their decision.

What's Up, Doc?

There are two kinds of Americans: Those who have spent time as a hospital patient, and those who are going to. We know these visits are likely to be lifesaving, but we'd like to postpone the pleasure as long as possible. When that day comes, for you or for a family member, here are some questions that can make your stay smoother and safer. Asking them can take away some of the anxiety induced by watching *Chicago Hope* reruns, and they can help avoid troublesome snafus once you're inside.

"A smooth hospital visit starts beforehand," says Karen N., the patient representative at a community hospital.

Here are a few of the questions you will want to ask: Ask the doctor, *What can I expect? Whom will I be meeting, and what will happen first? What tests will I be given? How long will I be there?*

"Many patients think the doctor is going to be right there to greet them when they come to the hospital," Karen says. "They're disappointed and scared; there's nobody they know."

"Even doctors with a small private practice don't hang out at the hospital," she points out.

Not only that, but if you belong to a health maintenance organization (HMO) or other big managed-care outfit, you may not see your doctor at the hospital at all. These groups have begun dividing their doctors into two groups: clinicians who see you for routine visits in their examining rooms, and "rounders," who make the rounds of all the hospital patients.

Who's in charge here? You need to know what physician will be coordinating your care. He or she is responsible for answering your basic questions and communicating your wishes about care. You may have a heavy traffic in doctors through your room. In theory, one of them is in charge. Find out whom? And, if nobody seems to be coordinating things, find out why. Many families face needless stress because they are meeting too many doctors who are not talking to each other. Be sure to ask, also, who will "cover" for the primary physician on weekends or during vacations. Many ethical disputes flare up when the covering physician isn't on the same page.

Who are these guys? You may feel like Butch Cassidy, pursued by a posse of nameless faces. You may be seen by several consultants. You have a right to know who the men and women are and what their roles are. (In a recent hospital experience, I was visited on successive days by three different cardiologists, each substituting for my "real" heart doctor. Each had opinions that varied just enough from the others to be unsettling.)

What's wrong with me? You have a right to know what your illness is and what the doctors think your chances are for full recovery. Incredibly, you have less than a fifty-fifty chance of getting this information unless you ask for it, clearly and assertively. There are still physicians who think too frank a discussion will endanger the patient, or that such information is too complex for laypeople. Others, believe it or not, prefer to tell relatives, and withhold the facts from the patient. If necessary, ask, and keep asking.

What's your plan? An ethically sensitive doctor will discuss the proposed treatment with you, including the risks and benefits and any alternate methods of treatment. If you're a member of a for-profit HMO, your doctor may be forbidden by contract to tell you about any courses of treatment not covered by the HMO. A more likely reason for withholding this information is that your doctor is afraid all the talk about side effects will freak you out.

Mind if I sit in? As one hospital's pamphlet for patients puts it, you have the right to "participate actively in decisions regarding medical care. This includes the right to refuse treatment."

Do you hear me squeaking? If you're having a problem and nobody seems to be listening, or if your decisions are being ignored, remember that the squeaky wheel gets the WD40. A hospital has many places to take your concern. Start with your primary (coordinating) physician, then the hospital patient representative or social worker. Any one of these might call a family conference, attended by your physicians, nurses, and any relatives you want present. Other helpful people are the head nurse, a chaplain, or even the hospital CEO's office. If your concern is ethical, ask for a meeting with members of the hospital's ethics (or bioethics) committee. Ethics committees don't hand down decisions. Better, they provide a forum for discussing all the angles of your problem. They'll support your rights as a patient.

One last word of advice. You may find these questions answered before you ask. Most doctors, nurses, and their colleagues in the hospital do an excellent job. But if not, remember that they are human, and appreciate a respectful approach and a kind word as much as the rest of us do.

Happy Anniversary

While Hurricane Harvey howled around us, winding down to a tropical storm again, we sat in a rented house on Fort Myers Beach and talked about death. No, not death from the storm; it was already clear from the incessant patter of the Weather Channel that Harvey had already done his worst. We talked about death, because we always have.

Death looked this family in the face before it got off the ground. Her doctor had advised Ma not to go through with the wedding. With his irregular heartbeat, Pa couldn't be expected to live more than a year. (A man born in the first decade of the century had a life expectancy of only 48.2 years anyway; a woman's was only 49.2.) She said she'd take her chances, and be grateful for whatever years they had. So, from the start they confronted death and its inevitability. Ma also talked about whether she wanted to marry a preacher, rather than suitors who seemed more likely to support her in style. She went with her heart.

A week after the wedding, the October stock crash started the Great Depression. For a young country pastor, death was part of the job. He sat with the families of men killed by their tractors and women cut down by cancer. Death snatched babies away before they had names.

The bishop sent Pa to a city church, but dealing with death didn't get any easier. In World War II, nineteen men from the congregation were in the armed services. In long talks and long silences, the pastor and his wife heard the deathly fears of those nineteen families, again and again. Five years after V-J Day, we were at war again. Pa drove miles out into the country to tell a mother that her only son would not be coming back from Korea.

Our family gatherings were hilarious and frequent, considering that at one time the three sons were living in Nigeria, Kenya, and Mississippi. Amidst the Yahtze and Pit games, somebody would remember the old hulk of a Chevy that we boys pushed into a prominent parking spot before church one Sunday. Ma would tell about using a hairpin to turn the ignition switch in the Model T Ford after the wedding, because the key was in Pa's other pants at home. During each reunion, Pa and Ma made it a point to get out the "Box" and go over the wills, the insurance papers, the instructions to the funeral home, the hymns to be sung at the memorial services. At first, we were uncomfortable with this. Who wants to talk with his parents about their deaths? But Ma and Pa had seen too many families unable and unprepared to deal with death as a natural part of life. They made their plans, and made sure we knew them.

They retired and moved to Florida, and after the first family gathering down there—their fortieth wedding anniversary—Pa said: "Well, I guess this is probably the last time we'll all be together." Despite our protests, we knew it could be true.

When the family gathered in California for their fiftieth wedding anniversary, Pa told about the first airplane he had ever seen flying low overhead: "My Dad said, 'Now, Vernon, don't you believe what you see. There's no man in that thing. It's a trick.' " Ma told about winding coils on a Baker's Chocolate box for Pa's homemade ham transmitter. When it was time to go back, Pa would say it: "Well, I suppose this is the last time I'll see you all. But it's been good."

At the sixtieth and sixty-fifth anniversaries, dominos and King in the Corner held sway. The brothers, once three-fourths of the college quartet, but now approaching retirement themselves, dusted off the old songs. The folks, in their high eighties, walked a mile before breakfast every day, and read widely. Ma was the greeter for new residents in the retirement home. By request, Pa was teaching a class on the Bible every Saturday. They stayed on their feet, mentally and physically.

And suddenly, it was September 1999, and time for a week-long celebration at Fort Myers Beach: the seventieth wedding anniversary. During the year, Ma had had two falls and a heart attack, but she was still on her feet, walking a half-mile, and beating us all at reminiscences. Pa had given up his class after seventy-five years of teaching. He had angina, but stayed in the thick of things.

The week on the beach was a success, divided between three days of the hurricane, and four of sunshine.

And we talked again of death as a fact of life.

Ma said, "I'm in no rush, but I'm ready when it's time."

Pa chuckled, "We might outlive all of you."

He was ninety-four, but we knew one of us could go first. My folks' legacy had been a firm faith, and a clear understanding that death is a part of life—for everybody.

Family Values

I guess you could call me a family values man—happily approaching a forty-eighth wedding anniversary as this is written, with four fine grown sons, and a brace of grandchildren. Since 1979, I've been working at the medical ethics trade—ethics being the study of values and how they are applied in daily life.

But, I can't for the life of me understand what the "family values" folks—the ones who claim to have a lock on the idea—are talking about. I thought it might help to get a list of values. A friend lent me a booklet called "Moral and Civic Education," put out by the state of California as a guide for schoolteachers. Published under a Republican governor, it had to please a panel that ranged from the retired admirals of San Diego to the public advocates of San Francisco. It affirms that the "American heritage and laws reflect a common core of personal and social morality," and began defining that core right on the first page: "Habits that reveal a commitment to moral values include telling the truth, being trustworthy, and respecting the opinions of others."

"Moral people affirm the worth and dignity of others in their attitudes and actions. They take responsibility for their decisions and for the consequences of those decisions. Moral people also value freedoms of conscience and respect the freedom of conscience of others."

What in the world? Can this be?

From my reading of the news, "family values" are about putting uppity women in their place. They are about forming a phalanx around a family planning clinic and screaming and shouting at women who already have enough troubles. And, on occasion, blowing up a clinic or two. Don't give me this "respect for freedom of conscience" baloney. I turn on the radio, and learn that my wife and many of our friends are "feminazis," bent on destroying families and castrating men. I learn that the rich are a downtrodden class, every one of whom has earned every cent but is victimized constantly by the greedy poor. Telling the truth? Affirming the worth and dignity of others? Forget it, pal; obviously, I was reading the wrong stuff.

I turn to the politicians, and learn that the M16 (which I understand is some sort of macho Rambo gun) is the cure of choice for the agony, longing, frustration, and violence of the ghetto. I learn that the untreated illnesses of millions of fellow Americans because they lack health insurance is regrettable but unavoidable, since no candidate is foolish enough to go head-to-head with the AMA, the hospital associations and the health insurance industry. Don't give me that business about "taking responsibility for their decisions and for the consequences of those decisions." And on all sides, I hear "family values" people, from right-wing preachers to state legislators, railing against bills that would ensure the rights of the Constitution for gay and lesbian people. In Oregon and Colorado, the FV folk actually led referendum campaigns to outlaw any such bill.

Aside from the fact that these may be the first measures taken by any state since Reconstruction to diminish the rights of a minority, these folks certainly show how wrong the values booklet must be when it suggests that "respect for differences is intrinsic to the healthy development of a heterogeneous society," and that "in a free society all persons and groups are to be treated equitably."

Obviously, California had it all wrong.

So I turned instead to the survey made last year for Massachusetts Mutual. Professional pollsters showed people across the country a list of values, and were asked which described a family value "very well." In first place, listed by 78 percent, was "being responsible for your actions." Second, 76 percent, was "respecting other people for who they are." Third was "being able to provide emotional support to your family."

Nah. Somebody else is to blame. Get rid of the queers. And don't bug me about pregnancy leave. Obviously, the American people are misinformed. They don't understand what family values are all about either.

A Noble Outcome

This wasn't going to be one of our duller Ethics Committee meetings. You could tell that when the Jack-in-the-box son began handing around printouts from the Internet. The patient. Marie K, seventy-four, first came to this hospital twelve years ago, for tests on a kidney. It was cancer, but the disease hadn't spread beyond the one kidney. It was removed surgically, and Mrs. K hadn't been near the hospital since. A few weeks ago, she came back. After twelve years of health, the remaining kidney was cancerous. This time there was no spare.

As Dr. H explained it to the patient and her daughters, the chemotherapy wasn't working. Mrs. K's best hope was removal of the second kidney, and a life of kidney dialysis three times a week. Mrs. K gave permission for the surgery, but before it could be scheduled, her body began saying, "no." She was sickly, losing weight. She developed pneumonia and needed help from a respirator to breathe. She had intravenous lines in her arms. The other organs began shutting down. Only the cancer was getting stronger. Mrs. K slipped into a deep sleep, and twenty-four hours later still hadn't awakened.

Dr. H talked with the surgeon, the cancer specialist, and the family doctor. They agreed that the cure-oriented plan no longer made sense. They would recommend a vigorous program aimed at making Mrs. K's remaining time peaceful and comfortable. Mrs. K's daughters agreed. But, a new face was now at the bedside—a son who lived 800 miles away and hadn't been heard from before. When he heard the doctors' recommendation, he was outraged.

"The last I heard, just before I left for the airport, was that Mom was doing fairly well—conscious, ready for surgery, and likely to live on for some time without pain. Now you're talking about letting her die!"

Everybody who works with dying patients recognizes Jack-(or Jill-) in-the-box. Eight times out of ten, the family member insisting on a full-court press is the one farthest removed—either geographically or emotionally—from the patient. That's not to say Jack had no right to speak up. The doctors heard his objections, and tried to explain their recommendations. But Jack just got more angry. When Dr. H emphasized again that the team had tried everything "appropriate," Jack began pulling more printouts from his flight bag. "Here's a treatment I learned about on the Internet. Have you tried this on Mom?"

No, Dr. H hadn't. "The Food and Drug Administration has been testing it for twenty years, without results. We have nothing more to suggest. I'm very sorry."

Jack was crying, half in anger, half in pain. "How can you just give up like that? Here's something that has saved lives."

The family physician interrupted, suggesting a family conference with members of the Ethics Committee the next day. By the time of the meeting, the caregivers were disagreeing among themselves.

Dr. K: "Even if this protocol isn't harmful, I can't recommend it. It could sidetrack energy from the comfort-care plan, possibly causing your mother more pain."

Dr. H (the family doctor): "Jack already has the pills. Couldn't we just look the other way as they administer them? That way they could feel they had tried everything."

Ms. Benton, R.N.: "It would put the nurses in a bind. It would violate federal law to give it in the hospital, or let it be given. We're responsible for every medication taken on our floor."

Ms. Jensen, social worker: "If the family cares for her at home, can they give her whatever medications they choose? Let's check it out."

Jack seemed calmer, and Dr. K more reasonable. Each family member talked at length, and the group adjourned.

Over the next few days, Jack and Dr. K spoke several times. The oncologist explained his need to be absolutely honest, even when it hurt. Even a partial lie would destroy trust, and leave the family with less hope, he felt. The turnaround came when Jack came to believe that the doctors' suggestions grew out of concern for his mother—not from a desire to enrich the hospital. Jack said he knew his mother was dying. He just wanted to be sure everything reasonable was being done. Now, he stopped pressing.

"You listened," he said.

His sister: "We still have hope. But it's a realistic hope, that Mom's time will be comfortable and peaceful. Who could wish for more than that?"

Durable Power of Attorney FAQs

Here are some of the questions most often asked about the Durable Power of Attorney for Health Care.

Q: What is it, and why should I care?

A: It's a simple legal document that gives you a continuing voice in your care, even if you're in a coma. Without it, doctors may have to guess at your wishes. Unfortunately, fewer than 25 percent of the people in a hospital on the day you're reading this have filled one out.

Q: How does it work?

A: The heart of the document is a paragraph in which you create a Power of Attorney (for health decisions only), and name a surrogate to speak for you. This "agent" will talk with the doctors and try to make the ethical decisions you would have made if you had been conscious. As your surrogate voice, your agent should be somebody who knows your opinions well.

Q: That's all there is to a DPAHC?

A: Those are the essentials; the rest varies from state to state. Many states provide space for you to write specific wishes as a guide to your agent, or check paragraphs that reflect your thinking. I chose not to use this feature in my DPAHC, and when I'm asked, I advise against it. The reason: It's impossible to foresee every dilemma, so it may be irrelevant when the crisis comes. Worse, in an unforeseen situation the sentences written out can be interpreted as exactly opposite to what the agent knows is your real wish; I've seen this happen more than once. The genius of the DPAHC (the abbreviation is usually pronounced "DEE-pack"), is in having an agent who knows your feelings and has your trust. They can ask questions of the doctor, or negotiate with her no matter what situation comes up.

Q: Does the DPAHC become effective when I sign it?

A: No. It becomes effective when you become comatose, or otherwise (as in advanced Alzheimer's disease) incapable of making decisions.

Q: Who determines whether I'm incapable or not?

A: Your attending physician, following widely accepted guidelines.

Q: What if I wake up?

A: You immediately resume your role as the person who gives or withholds consent for all medical treatment. In most states, by the way, the DPAHC has no expiration date. But you can revoke it by voice any time you choose.

Q: Can I name both my daughters as agents?

A: No, but you can name one as agent and the other as first alternate—and assume they get along. Remember that your agent is the one person with legal power to speak for you.

Q: Can I just write out a "living will" that states my wishes in specific situations?

A: Yes, but the odds are against your foreseeing every possible situation. Then your relatives and the doctors are back to guessing. Your DPAHC agent can face an unexpected situation, ask questions of the caregivers, and decide the real issue, in real time.

Q: Do I need a lawyer?

A: No, just two witnesses. If you don't have two friends who fit the requirements for witnesses, one notary public can sign, seal and deliver.

Q: What if I'm injured in another state?

A: Your DPAHC won't be a legal document there, backed by a law in the same sense as it is in your home state. But a signed statement naming somebody to make decisions for you, and possibly spelling out some specifics, can't hurt when it comes to making tough health care decisions anywhere.

Q: Where do I get one of these forms?

A: Your doctor should have them. Your hospital not only has them, but will help you complete one if you haven't already.

Q: Who should keep my copy?

A: Make that plural. Make photocopies and give them to your physician, your rabbi, priest or pastor; your lawyer; every close relative, and close friends. Keep one with you.

Q: What if I have doctors who hint they won't follow my wishes?

A. Dump them. Informed patient consent is the law, and a DPAHC is just one way to protect that right. Doctors who in good conscience can't go along with your wishes should help you transfer care to a doctor who will.

Q: Can you guarantee that it will work?

A: No. There are still doctors who ignore or flout a patient's wishes. But, your chances of being heard are much better when a legal surrogate, backed by this document, stands up for your rights.

Ethical Goals

Everybody knows that a good bit of our health care dollar is spent on older and dying patients. What we're not sure about are these two questions:

- Just how much, exactly?
- Is it something we should get in an uproar about?

The figures you hear on the street range from 25 percent to 90 percent. One man said in conversation, "Do you know that half of all our health care money is eaten up in the last six months of people's lives?" A few days earlier, somebody else had said, "We use up 75 percent of the Medicare money on dying people hooked up to those machines." There have been half a dozen such conversations recently; we're all talking a lot of health care these days. Each time the figure was different, but pronounced with authority. One thing was consistent, though—each time, there was a "therefore." For example:

"People over seventy shouldn't be put on life support."

"Older people should just be allowed to die naturally, without all this high-tech stuff."

"There should be a law against these old folks using up all the health care money."

My ears were especially tuned to all this folk wisdom, because I had rediscovered, in what passes for my files, a golden oldie article from a medical journal, one of my favorites. Although it was published several years ago, the figures it gave are still good; and most of the changes it called for are happening. The article in the *New England Journal of Medicine* was called, "The Care of the Terminally Ill: Morality and Economics." The date was Dec. 15, 1983. The authors pointed out that the usual dilemmas surrounding death in the ICU were becoming "even more complex because of a growing, if ill-defined, economic concern that often lurks just below the surface of recent discussions. . . . Terminal care often involves intensive and expensive treatment, and questions have been raised about its value. Is the cost too high? Is it 'wasteful'?"

The article cited several studies of the expenses of dying. One study found that more than 20 percent of the expenses in private, non-psychiatric hospitals were for the terminally ill. Another looked at what percent of all the people enrolled in Medicare died in a given year: 5 percent. Then it totaled up how much of the Medicare money was spent on those patients in that year: 22 percent.

The Health Care Financing Administration told one set of researchers that terminal care accounted for 19 to 22 percent of all Medicare reimbursements, and that the figure remains constant over several years.

So, for purposes of your next discussion, a good round 20 percent is a figure you can back up. (There's another intriguing way to put it: In hospitals, the total care per patient of those who die is usually double the care of those who survive to go home.) Settling the factual question doesn't make the ethical one any easier. If we know that one-fifth of the billions we spend on health care is spent during the last act, what does that mean? Does it mean, as a whole gaggle of Beamers have suggested, that the oldsters are unfairly robbing them of money that is justly theirs? Are these figures ammunition for yet another war of the generations? Does it mean that care should be more heavily rationed for the elderly? That—as one pundit suggested—patients over eighty-five should have comfort care only; no high-tech "rescues"?

The authors of the 1983 article suggested concentrating on three other goals: Each goal is not only ethically acceptable, but saves money.

- Develop better criteria for admission to the intensive care unit and critical-care wards. In the past, doctors sent the very sick to these wards. Now they're asking, "What are the odds of this patient's getting better?" "Will this patient survive the ICU?" An example is a person who suffers a heart attack on the street and is unable to be resuscitated there or in the ambulance. The odds are less than 1 percent of living to leave the hospital. Doctors today are much less likely to incur the $1,000 to $3,000 a day expense of virtually useless treatment.
- Promote patient and family autonomy in decisions to stop or refuse certain kinds of treatment. It has been interesting to see an about-face among hospital administrators on this issue. Ten years ago, they were afraid to have doctors withhold treatment, for fear of lawsuits. Now—either because it's clearly the ethical thing to do, or because it saves the hospital money—they listen when the patient refuses treatment.
- Promote alternate care, including hospice care. The human value of the dedicated staff and volunteers in hospice, who devote themselves to comforting the dying, is widely known. And, there's a growing awareness of the values in home care, even for the dying. It worked for thousands of years, and may be an idea whose time has come   again.

To Tell the Truth

Must physicians always tell the truth, the whole truth, and nothing but the truth? Or, are there times when a little white lie is actually in the patient's interest? The question comes up again because of the beating the truth seems to be taking elsewhere. Cover-ups, character attacks, and the swoosh of hot air from political spins make us wonder what the truth is. And worse, to ask whether it really matters anymore. Well, one person to whom it matters is Harvard professor Sissela Bok.

She's one of the world's true experts on equivocation, a professor of prevarication, if you will.

Her book on the subject brought high praise when it was published twenty years ago and is still selling well in paperback. In keeping with her no-nonsense approach, the book is simply called, *Lying*. A teacher of ethics at the Harvard Medical School, Bok got into the subject of lying while doing research for a medical journal article on placebos— the sugar pills doctors sometimes give patients for their psychological effect. Soon she had run into numerous other situations involving white lies and white coats.

Should a physician lie to dying patients so as to delay the fear and anxiety which the truth might bring them? Should a doctor lie to a patient to avoid worry that might delay his or her recovery? Bok found a widely known Catholic medical textbook that advised doctors and nurses to lie "by mental reservation" when they thought it was wise to do so. She writes: "If a feverish patient, for example, asks what his temperature is, the doctor is advised to answer, 'Your temperature is normal today,' while making the mental reservation that it is normal for someone in the patient's precise physical condition."

A physician was asked by a long-time patient to certify that "medical reasons" made it unwise to bus her seven-year-old boy into another neighborhood as part of a court-ordered racial integration program. Family members whose "spare" kidney is a life-saving match for a patient sometimes agree to be a donor while hiding deep anxieties and a strong desire not to donate. Physicians who recognize such a situation will sometimes honor the unwilling donor's unexpressed wishes by reporting falsely that he or she was not a good tissue match. For example, genetic tests for newborn babies, developed in the last decade, can reveal that the husband is not the baby's father. Must the doctor tell? In Oregon, the new law allowing physician-assisted suicide (PAS) has created truth-telling dilemmas. Doctors are not required to participate in

PAS if it violates their conscience, but are required, as in all medical procedures, to refer the patient to another physician. But they are not required by law to tell the patient about PAS while discussing end-of-life care. Do they have a moral duty to tell, when not telling limits the choices of the patient?

Bok made two daunting discoveries while researching her book. First, she found, "[The] requirement to be honest with patients has been left out altogether from medical oaths and codes of ethics, and is often ignored, if not actually disparaged, in the teaching of medicine." Doctors want the option of lying left open, Bok found, because of "a severely restricted and narrowed paternalistic view—that some patients cannot understand, some do not want, and some may be harmed by knowledge of their condition."

Second, ". . . many physicians talk about such deception in a cavalier, often condescending and joking way, whereas patients often have an acute sense of injury and of loss of trust at learning that they have been duped." This is an outgrowth of the old paternalistic model of medical practice, in which the doctor is the lord of the castle, up on the hill, and the patient is the village idiot down in the flatlands.

Both these situations have changed since *Lying* was first published. Many medical schools now have ethics courses, and truth-telling is stressed. Most physicians consider truth-telling an important ideal—although many still find rationalization for the "therapeutic lie." The burden of proof has to fall increasingly on the physician who wants to bend the truth; it can't any longer be done casually or condescendingly. Bok offers three reasons for telling patients the truth:

- ". . . The medical and psychological benefits to them from this knowledge.
- "The unnecessary and sometimes harmful treatment to which they can be subjected if ignorant,
- "[And] the harm to physicians, their profession, and other patients. . . ."

Part Two | Alternative Reproductive Technology

eOva

They breed horses, don't they? Why not people?

That, in a nutshell, is the rationale for a movement called eugenics—the hope that things will get better if we can just breed a better strain of human babies. One of the latest gurus to promote the idea is Los Angeles fashion photographer Ron Harris, who has used the Internet to auction off ova, or eggs, from some of his most beautiful models. Harris says five million people hit on www.ronsangels.com the first half-day it was online. What they got was a set of three pictures and an editorial. The three faces shown could be described as (left to right) wholesome, sultry, and perky. Net surfers who have been unable to have a baby were invited to make a choice, then bid for a cluster of ova from their favorite. The written matter demonstrated that eugenics—not infertility—is Harris's main concern. He writes of "millions of men from around the world who would love to have their genes combined with the most beautiful women. Many men have substantial financial resources, yet are unable to find the genetic combinations that would impart beauty to their offspring." Noting proudly that he has "developed several theories about biology and beauty," he offers this one: "Choosing eggs from beautiful women will profoundly increase the success of your children and your children's children, for centuries to come. Any gift such as beauty, intelligence or social skills will help your children in their quest for happiness and success."

Who could resist such an offer?

Unfortunately, those most passionate about eugenics seem to have had better grounding in media relations than in the science of genetics. The guy who set up a sperm bank with deposits from Nobel prize winners in the 1980s had a Nobel himself—but his field was transistors, not genetics. His act flopped. Harris's qualifications seem to be a photographic eye and experience in breeding Arabian horses. One of the best-known eugenics zealots was Adolf Hitler, who used concentration-camp inmates as unwilling subjects for experiments aimed at strengthening and purifying the "Aryan race."

Americans were swept up in the movement in the mid-1920s, when well-intentioned geneticists acted on faulty data: studies that seemed to show that immigrants from northern Europe were more self-reliant and industrious than those from southern Europe. They successfully lobbied Congress for a drastic cut in the number of U.S. immigrants from the south of Europe. The quota of Greeks, for example, was chopped from 64,000 a year to 64 a year. By the time the bad science was exposed, great harm had been done to many thousands of would-be Americans.

The ova-on-auction (eOva?) may just be a gag. Harris admits that among the first five million hits, there were only five bids—one of which seemed sincere. But suppose he's serious. What's wrong with getting infertile people together with the best possible virtual mate? Here are a few of the things that worry ethicists and geneticists:

He can't deliver. The implication that the right genes can guarantee a "beautiful" child is a scam, an exploitation of our society's naive belief in "improving the breed."

He's making humanity a commodity. The powerful infertility industry has managed to avoid most federal regulation; Ova and sperm have escaped the federal ban on selling body parts for transplant. But the result is still dehumanizing. For this reason, the eBay auction Web site refuses to allow auctions of ova or sperm.

To be fair, we have to remember that Ron Harris didn't start this trend. The hot competition between fertility clinics has been doing this for several years. One Virginia clinic boasts on its extensive Web site: "We have recruited over 100 currently accessible egg donors meeting the highest medical and genetic screening standards." Another medical infertility clinic mails out an illustrated catalog of donors. The women are paid from $2,500 to $5,000. Except for the amounts, how is this different? By the way, couples who act fast can get a $1,000 discount on the procedure, which can cost $40,000.

Beauty is more mind and soul than physiognomy and measurements, and as the fella said, it's in the eye of the beholder. Anyway, one of those half-serious sociology studies found that men wanted three things in a woman: youth, beauty, and social skills. But when the pollsters asked women who seemed to fit those categories what they wanted in a man, the top three were good looks, youth, and lots of money.

Technology is outracing our wisdom. A few decades ago, there was a thirty-year gap between a scientific breakthrough and its application in daily life. That lead time is gone. We need to ask whether it makes sense to let the infertility industry and its lobbyists write their own rules while we play money games with the very stuff of human life.

Interim Septuplets

"Location, location, location," the real estate agent says. "Location is everything."

And now, says the Supreme Court, location may also be a crucial principle of medical ethics. You may have thought you'd heard the last of the divorced Tennessee couple fighting over their seven frozen embryos. But no, the case inched its way up the appeals ladder, through the Tennessee Supreme Court and finally, to a decision by the Supreme Court of the United States. It all began in 1988 in Knoxville, Tennessee, with a last-chance attempt by Mary Sue Davis and her husband, Junior Davis, to have a child. After all other methods had been tried, doctors at the Fertility Center of East Tennessee drew several eggs from her ovaries and put them with his sperm in a laboratory dish. The result was seven embryos, each about the size of the period at the end of this sentence. But before the doctor could implant one or two of them in Mary Sue's womb, the Davis's stressful marriage blew up. The couple separated, and the fertility clinic put the embryos on hold, immersing them in liquid nitrogen at some 300 degrees below zero. The two filed for divorce, but didn't have much trouble dividing the property—until it came to the embryos. Mary Sue wanted custody, saying she still wanted to use the embryos to get pregnant.

Junior said he no longer wanted to cooperate with Mary Sue on anything, and especially didn't want to father her baby. Mary Sue went to court, seeking custody; Junior asked that the embryos be destroyed. Judge W. Dale Young ruled that human life begins at conception, and therefore the seven dots were human beings, not property. He gave Mary Sue custody. Junior appealed, and the higher court reversed Young's ruling. It was Mary Sue's turn to appeal, but the Tennessee Supreme Court agreed with the appeals court, saying embryos may not be just property, but they aren't human beings either. It said they "occupy an interim category that entitles them to special respect because of their potential for human life." The Tennessee justices said Junior's right not to procreate overrode Mary Sue's right to have a child.

That was the decision the U.S. Supreme Court affirmed, by refusing to overturn it.

They didn't comment, but, here are some of the things they seemed to imply:

Location is crucial. The U.S. court had approved, without much enthusiasm, the principle in the 1973 *Roe v. Wade* decision: that the fate of an embryo/fetus in the first six months of pregnancy is a private matter between the mother-to-be and her doctor. Now, we wonder: does this apply only to embryos within the mother-to-be's body? Is, in this case, possession seven points of the law? Mary Sue Davis's embryos were not in her body, but in Knoxville, 15 miles up U.S. 129 from the couple's home. Their fate, the court said, was not in her hands alone.

Men, like women, may have a right not to procreate. Roe v. Wade said nobody, including the father to be and the government, could force a woman to continue a pregnancy. The court in this case seemed to be affirming this right for men as well.

Human life doesn't begin at the moment of fertilization—the instant when the sperm penetrates the egg. This conservative court, this basically anti-abortion court, might have been expected to affirm the belief, so crucial to the anti-abortion stand, that life begins with fertilization.

A strong and passionate minority in the United States has been working toward a constitutional amendment that would grant the full rights of humanhood to embryos from the moment of conception. Does the Supreme Court's science mean the justices don't buy this idea anymore?

Mary Sue, now remarried and living in Florida, still believes the embryos are children, and her lawyer says she's planning another way to get them back. Junior says a court will order them destroyed. And the head of the fertility clinic says he'd be unhappy doing that. Which means, after several years and four courts, we still may not have heard the last of Mary Sue, Junior, and the seven little beings in their cold and silent sleep.

Dead

Her world was the tubes and wires of the intensive-care unit, giving fluids or taking them away, monitoring her breathing and the steady beat of her heart. Another set of wires kept track of the second heart, the one in her womb. Outside the gray curtain drawn around her bed, the world was talking about Marie Odette Henderson—the woman who had died, but held within her a living fetus.

Marie Henderson has been in the grave now for several years. Her daughter is almost old enough for first grade. But, our understanding of the matters of life and death, and how we draw the lines, hasn't grown that much. Our confusion is pretty much as it was when these reports— all inaccurate—were reaching us from the hospital in Oakland:

CBS: "Marie Odette Henderson died today. She had been on life support since being pronounced brain-dead seven-and-a-half weeks ago."

San Francisco Chronicle: Henderson "is being kept alive through heroic efforts."

ABC-TV: Henderson is "in irreversible coma."

It wasn't the reporters' fault. Even doctors were—and are—confused by the new medical devices that blur the reliable old signs that death has occurred. It used to be simple. Doc Adams held a mirror to the nose of the unconscious, wounded Marshal Dillon and said, "He's alive; steam on the mirror shows he's breathing." Seventy-five years later Marcus Welby held a stethoscope to the chest of an accident victim and said, "Her heartbeat is weak, but it's there. She's alive." No breathing. A silent heart. Those have been the signs of death.

And those signs worked fine until the invention of the machine to which Henderson was attached: the artificial ventilator. With air pushed into the lungs, and medical adjustment of things like blood pressure and blood gases, the heart could keep pumping long after the brain had stopped telling it to. But, if the "vital signs" were normal, how did you know whether the patient was alive? A second breakthrough—the organ transplant—made it urgent to find an answer. Nobody wanted to take a kidney from a patient who was still alive.

Doctors, researchers, ethicists, and legislators eventually agreed on a new legal sign of death: the permanent absence of any brain activity. This definition is now part of the law of every state, and was the definition the doctors used when they pronounced Henderson dead in April 1986. Not "brain-dead." Not "lung-dead." They pronounced her dead. "There's no separate category of brain death," the president's commission on ethical problems in medicine said in a report. "Death is death."

But look at the confusion. On *life* support since being pronounced brain *dead*. "Kept alive . . ." "In a coma . . . ."

It's much more than semantics. This particular misunderstanding has caused as much pain for families and physicians as any other in the world of medicine. Two doctors were falsely (and successfully) charged with murder in Los Angeles; the source was confusion over the difference between "dead" and "in an irreversible coma." I know a hospital where the corpse of a little boy is being kept breathing by machines in a ghastly charade—simply because a doctor wanted to break the news gently to the family and told them the child was "in a coma." Now, the family's threat to sue keeps the hospital from doing what the law says should have been done in the first place—pronounce the boy dead, and remove the respirator along with the rest of the now-useless paraphernalia. If it really had been a coma, the boy would have looked exactly the same to a casual observer. But, there would have been a last remnant of brain activity. Legally, he would be a dying patient, not a dead one, and the respirator would truly be "life support."

The agony of the family and the health care team goes on—as it did for Marie Odette Henderson's loved ones until the baby was born, almost three months after Henderson had died.

Wistfully, a spokesman for the president's commission said around that time that public understanding of this whole subject "would be greatly aided" if the phrase "brain-dead" were never used, and if "mechanical ventilators were not called 'life support systems' when applied to dead bodies."

Considering the fact that 70 percent of hospital deaths now involve the decision to withdraw some kind of support, you'd think we'd want to get it straight.

The Littlest Preemie

It is one of the toughest ethics calls in medicine: "How hard should we struggle to save the life of this premature baby?" In an issue of the *New England Journal of Medicine,* researchers make the call a little easier. But, they also demonstrate how hard it is to make ethics decisions by the numbers. The major problem with low-birthweight babies is this: Fetuses are supposed to stay in the womb around thirty-seven weeks, each week bringing them closer to the full development needed to live outside. A baby born at, say, twenty-three weeks may still have a hole in its heart—a condition necessary for living in amniotic fluid, but life-threatening for a baby struggling to breathe air. In a normal pregnancy, the hole closes before birth. The lungs of a twenty-three-week baby may still be sealed against the fluid in the womb, not opened up for oxygen. Its skull may still be so soft that its brain can be damaged during the birth process. Many other changes take place in the last three months. So, the earlier the baby is born, the more likely it is to have serious birth defects, some of them potentially fatal. Technology has been making it possible to keep these little tykes alive earlier and earlier, with miniature respirators, tube feeding, and microsurgery. But many of those who survive will die a few months later anyway. Others may live on for years, but with chronic illness, retardation, or physical disabilities.

The second problem is this: The Supreme Court has ruled that only the patient in question can know whether the quality of life is good enough to continue treatment. If the patient were an adult, we would have some idea of how he or she would have answered the question. But we can't ask the preemie. In the end, the parents and the doctors share the terrible choice. The new research, conducted at Johns Hopkins medical school, narrows the choice. Studying 142 low-birthweight babies—all of whom would have died before the current technology was developed—the researchers found that babies born after twenty-five weeks of pregnancy survived without major birth defects. But those born before twenty-two weeks of pregnancy, the researchers found, are probably doomed no matter how hard the doctors and nurses fight on their behalf. None of the Johns Hopkins babies born at less than 22 weeks survived as much as six weeks. So the new research simplified the question a little.

In the "should" and "ought" language of ethics, every effort probably should be made to save babies born at twenty-five weeks or more. The burden—cost of treatment, involvement of large staffs of nurses and doctors—is outweighed in most people's minds by the benefit: a healthy child. Weighing burden versus benefit for the twenty-two-week low-birthweight baby, most people would question the value of intense treatment. The baby's chance of survival is close to zero. The dilemma is in between; the researchers have left us with that gap between twenty-two and twenty-five weeks. Consider life span in the Johns Hopkins study: Of those born after a twenty-three-week pregnancy, 85 percent died before six months; at twenty-four weeks, forty-four percent; at twenty-five weeks, 21 percent. Odds short enough, in each case, to lean either way. Or, consider the quality of life: 98 percent of those born at twenty-three weeks of pregnancy had severe abnormalities; at twenty-four weeks it was 79 percent, and at twenty-five weeks, still 31 percent.

The "burden" here is more than cash, although treating one of these babies can cost anywhere from $350,000 to $500,000. Another burden is that of the parents—modifying the house for a disabled child; the effect on other children of the special attention that must be given, often indefinitely, to the patient; the emotional impact on the marriage, which in many cases doesn't survive; the societal cost of schooling and care. The heaviest burden—or greatest benefit—is that of the patient, the child. Will he or she say someday, "I wish I hadn't been born" (as nineteen of twenty spina bifida patients in wheelchairs, paralyzed from the shoulders down, told researchers in another study). Or will he or she be one of those rare but shining lives who overcome all odds, to shed love and joy wherever they are? It's a heavy question, an unanswerable one that demands sympathy—not judgment—for all parents and professionals who face it.

To Be a Mother

A bioethics question argued (a few years ago) from Spain to Australia, was not just who is a mom, but who *ought* to be one. According to reports, Italy, Australia, Spain, Sweden, and the United Kingdom are all embroiled in debates over the new reproduction. Most of the cases involve *in vitro* fertilization (IVF), the technique by which a human ovum or egg is fertilized outside the body and then implanted to start a pregnancy. It's not a new idea. Thousands of infertile couples have used it, but there has always been a low-key debate, kept alive by those who question the morality of the whole procedure.

Now comes a different criticism: It may be all right, but only for certain women. It's a "moral" test, not a biological one. Consider some of the cases reported in recent years:

Australia—This story could have been one of those heartwarmers. Two women, made infertile by ovarian cancer, getting a chance to have babies after all. Before their cancer therapy, eggs were removed from the ovaries of each woman and frozen by a newly refined procedure developed by Dr. Debra Gook. The plan was for the eggs to be thawed and fertilized and the resulting embryos to be implanted after the cancer treatment was over. Just one problem: The law in the state of Victoria forbids IVF in women who are single or lesbian. Dr. Gook, a biochemist at the Royal Women's Hospital, told Reuters, "It's unbelievable. It's quite ridiculous. We're not doing crazy, brave new world type of stuff." The state says if the two women want to find men to marry, then they can take advantage of the new science. Under pressure, a spokesman said last week the state might consider letting unmarried women use the procedure—if they were in a stable relationship.

Italy—After a year of deliberation, the National Committee for Bioethics brought in its recommendations, without surprising anybody. It said artificial pregnancy should be available only to "adult couples of different sex who are married or at least bound by a stable and loving relationship and . . . preferably are of a potentially fertile age." In the absence of laws, Italian doctors had used IVF to impregnate women in their sixties, women in same-sex relationships, and in one case, a black woman with a white baby. This aroused a fuss that some observers suggested was as much related to ageism, racism, and homophobia as to technology. Like a booster rocket for the debate was the birth of a baby girl to a lesbian couple, just three days before release of the report. The mother had been artificially inseminated by sperm from a donor bank, and the doctor came under heavy criticism. Parliament is expected to turn the committee's recommendations, which have church backing, into law.

Spain—Spain is different; a five-year-old law makes IVF and artificial insemination available to all women—not just those in couples. But Spain has a problem with leftovers. The IVF process draws out and fertilizes anywhere from eight to thirty eggs—far more than are needed. In Spain, these embryos, which some people consider full human beings, are frozen and, after two years, are available for use by other infertile women. But fertility clinics don't usually make them available; they're afraid the donors might show up some day to claim them, and sue if they're gone. At the heart of the dilemma is the fact that the 1988 law authorized a national bioethics committee to deal with such questions—but the committee has never been formed.

Sweden finally dealt—sort of—with a related problem: Who's a daddy? A Swedish woman had impregnated herself with sperm given her in a hotel lobby by a Danish man, and recently sought child support for her little boy, now three years old. But a Stockholm court ruled in late June that since they never had sexual intercourse, and weren't in a long-term relationship, the Dane was not legally a father.

United Kingdom—A Manchester judge set a precedent when he recognized a twenty-two-month-old boy as having two mothers. At the request of a young lesbian couple, identified only as Debbie and Julie, he granted full custody and parental responsibility to both women, making Julie as much a mom under the law as Debbie, the biological mother.

Genome Dilemmas

"They took a picture of the baby and I know what it is," she said as soon as her husband picked up the telephone. "Would you like to know?"

"No!" he said. "I thought we agreed that we didn't want to know till it's born. What if they got it wrong?"

"Oh, I know we agreed. But, the doctor was taking the sonogram anyway, and she said the fetus was just in perfect position for us to see whether it's going to be a boy or girl. I even have a little snapshot of it. Sure you don't want to see?"

As you read this, somebody not too far away is happily sharing the results of her sonogram, or amniocentesis, or some other high-tech peek into the watery world of a little curled-up human-to-be. Most of the time, it's an occasion for joy, and the decision about whether the parents really want to know the baby's sex isn't a heavy one. But as science develops more and better windows into the womb, the decision about whether we really want to know everything is getting harder—and the ethical consequences heavier. For example, the ability to test, in the womb or in early childhood, for genes that increase the likelihood of getting cancer or heart disease. It's information that could save a life—or make the person permanently unemployable.

The potential for trouble is great enough that the National Center for Genome Research and the National Cancer Institute held a three-day conference just to talk about the ethical dilemmas. The genome center has a fifteen-year program to explore the hundreds of thousands of genes in the center of each cell of the human body. Some of these genes have a direct effect; if you're born with the gene for Tay-Sachs disease, for example, you will die from that cruel malady, probably before you're a year old. Genes for cystic fibrosis and dozens of other inherited diseases are equally predictable: you have the gene, you have the illness.

There is no cure. The obstetrician can find out, early in pregnancy, whether the gene is there; if it is, the parents-to-be must struggle with the moral question of whether to continue the pregnancy.

But research in and out of the genome project is identifying a different kind of gene, one that adds to the moral dilemma. This kind of gene predisposes you to a specific disease. It increases your risk. But it's not certain that you'll contract the problem at all. An example is a gene, BRCA1, that raises the odds of a woman's getting breast cancer sometime in her life to as high as 80 percent. But 20 percent will never be afflicted. Another gene is responsible for 85 percent of all cases of kidney cancer. More than 23,000 people each year come down with new cases of this cancer—but 15 percent of the people carrying that gene are not afflicted. Since health care costs are so high, many big employers are asking would-be employees to take a genetic test for genes that might—just might—cause cancer or heart disease. Hiring such a person could send the employer's insurance costs sky-high.

Surveys indicate that more than a hundred of the Fortune 500 companies are doing some of this testing now. Many life insurance and health insurance companies are also testing for these iffy genes. After all, if they insured the people most likely to get sick, there would be no profits. But what about the patient, the would-be worker, the applicant for insurance? The odds are strong that the Misfortune 100 are already turning down people who are not sick, and who never will contract the cancer or heart disease they're at risk for. And, in the future, such people—many of them perfectly healthy—could be permanently unemployable as health risks.

Now, some of this will change. Pressure from the Clinton proposals has already caused some insurance companies to stop the practice of dropping anybody off the roll if he or she is likely to get sick. Congress seems to be serious about making the health insurance industry actually live up to its name. And, when there is universal coverage (if there ever is), spreading the risk across a wider base, employers won't have to worry about being bankrupted by high-cost, high-visibility illnesses. Until then, doctors will have to struggle over what's right. Should they urge the patient to take the test, with the possibility of bad consequences outweighing the good? Should they take the time to talk over all the issues with the patient, at the cost of time for other patients? Do these genes, found in families, require a new ethic in which the doctor tells other family members about the discovery? How should doctors interpret the odds? Should a young woman with the gene that gives her an 80 percent chance of getting ovarian and breast cancer have her ovaries and breasts removed? And would it be better not to know? Who can say?

When I'm 64

What bothers us so much about the sixty-three-year-old woman who recently became a mother? Around office coffeepots, reactions range from uneasy to indignant. The talking heads at six and ten o'clock, for lack of something better to say, drone on about "raising ethical issues," but don't actually mention any.

Nobody suggests a baby shower.

Why are we so troubled? What pushed our button? The news coverage is not the kind we get about the oldest woman in the county. Those stories are fondly approving. We applaud the one-hundred-year-old, whether she deserves the credit for the feat or not. But, a mother who's nearly sixty-four! Instead of congratulations, the stories say "tsk tsk!" And the emotion is so universal, nobody is asking, "What are we afraid of?"

Is it the technology that so repels us? Hardly. We love that stuff. Look at the recent hoo-hah over a half-baked idea like cloning. We watch developments with a sort of delicious dread—not the outrage we bring to the aging-mom stories. The technology is safe and simple. Her husband's sperm fertilized a donor egg in the lab and the microscopic embryo was implanted in her womb. A sixty-two-year-old Italian woman became a mother the same way in 1994, and the general fuss was the same. Around the world, people didn't like it.

Is it our concern for the child, then? Many worry about the mother's being seventy-six when her daughter hits the teens, or leaving her an orphan before she's grown. But come on, folks, get real. Hundreds of thousands of kids are being raised by their grandmothers. But there's no movement to outlaw these arrangements. There is only sporadic national discussion. The feeling seems to be that grannies may have less energy, but more wisdom than when they were younger. The possibility of one orphan is raising more dust than the existence of millions of orphans in refugee camps.

No, there's something more. I'm convinced that we are so spooked because the aging mother challenges barriers we have set up for women—especially older women. She's out of her territory, threatening walls built centuries ago. The Greeks taught us to think of the mind and body as separate. Mind was good, body evil. Mind was rational; body was emotional. Mind was male, body was female. The Church called this a heresy, but embraced some of it anyway. Gradually, sex and the body came to be seen as necessary evils whose only value was in procreation. Having thus segregated women theologically, history went on to divide their lives sharply into four phases, each with strict rules for behavior: child, maiden, mother, and old woman. Only one of these phases was supposed to have anything to do with sex, and that only because children were necessary. It was grudgingly conceded that the newly married woman had a sexual side. But when childbearing duties were completed, a good woman was supposed to lapse back into asexuality. This had little to do with reality, of course. But, it had everything to do with defining and controlling women's lives.

The anonymous California woman who became a mother at sixty-three years and nine months has violated our centuries-old expectations of womanly behavior. She became a mother when she was supposed to be on the sidelines. Nothing else explains the strong emotions she has raised in the rest of us. We resent her because of sexism and ageism, buried so deep in our psyches we don't recognize how they trigger our emotions. An example of how this can work: A college professor I knew in the 1960s was teaching a course on sexuality. One day, after seeing part of a film showing a couple making love, the class rebelled and walked out on him. It wasn't the subject; he'd shown such films before. This time, however, the married couple in the movie were in their sixties. The twenty-something students couldn't deal with it. Thousands of years of ageist history is trying to tell us there is no place at the center for a woman nearly sixty-four years old. She's supposed to shuffle off into the background, making way for the young and active.

47

Anybody who challenges that kind of pigeonholing, who dares to live richly outside the stereotype, should expect to find the world fidgety and disapproving.

Let's hope that this continues to change. In the meantime, we need to be curious about why our knee jerks, and not be surprised when the singer asks, "Will you still need me, will you still feed me, when I'm sixty-four?"

Advances in the Test Tube

One thing Doctors R. G. Edwards and Patrick Steptoe never foresaw, as they worked to fertilize a human egg in the lab, was that they would also give birth to a $2 billion cutthroat industry. Edwards, the scientist, and Steptoe, the obstetrician, thought they could help the 25 percent of infertile women whose problem was an obstruction in their fallopian tubes, keeping egg and sperm from meeting naturally. By 1975, they had implanted more than 100 women with the pinhead-sized embryos created in the lab from the wife's egg and the husband's sperm. It was *in vitro* fertilization (IVF), because it was done "in glass" rather than in the body. It would be another three years before they introduced the world's first child conceived in a laboratory dish. Her name was Louise Brown.

Meanwhile, the IVF industry was expanding like a birthday balloon. By 1985, 30 U.S. fertility clinics were using *in vitro* techniques, and reported 260 babies that year. By 1994, there were more than 300 clinics, and they reported, 12,463 IVF babies. The competition was fierce because desperate couples would pay just about any amount you asked. IVF was the last word in high-tech medicine, and the last resort for childless couples who wanted babies. Results and rates: that was the draw. The fertility clinic with the best ratio of delivered babies to enrolled patients, at the lowest cost, would get more of the business. The pie they were cutting up totaled $2 billion a year.

Pressure came from the fact that fewer than 20 percent of their IVF clients get pregnant on each try. At $10,000 or more per attempt, the price could easily run $50,000 or more. Some couples felt they weren't told the whole story up front—the low rates of success and the risks to the fetuses, for example. Even some obvious no-nos were perpetrated by a few. A fertility specialist at the University of California-Irvine, for example, was accused of stealing extra ova from some of his healthier patients, then fertilizing and implanting them in other women. It helped his success rate. In 1992, a Virginia specialist was convicted of fraud and perjury for using his own sperm to father at least seventy children in the lab. He saved on donor fees, and reported a creditable success rate.

Most labs play it straight. But all of them practice one procedure that is ethically questionable. They implant three or more embryos at each attempt, hoping at least one will thrive and grow to babyhood. That helps bring down the price, and ups their success rate. But sometimes *all* the embryos grow, as the McCaughey septuplets demonstrated. This use of multiple embryos is the major reason for a 25 percent increase in the birth of twins in the United Kingdom between 1980 and 1993. During the same thirteen years, the rate of triplets and quadruplets doubled. That rise, echoed in the United States and Canada, might be okay if the only side effect of multiple births were cute costumes and a heavy traffic in diapers.

But as we've pointed out before, there is a dark side to multiple births. Kids born three or more at a time have a greater risk of the mental and physical defects that accompany incomplete gestation. They have a higher death rate. Thus the fertility specialist, deliberately implanting extra embryos, does so with the knowledge that some of the growing fetuses will be stillborn or seriously disabled. Some will be aborted, in the procedure called "selective reduction," in order to save the others. Recently, the *New England Journal of Medicine* joined the calls for "greater efforts . . . to decrease the rate of multiple pregnancies after assisted reproduction, because there is an increase in obstetrical complications." The one way to do this is by implanting fewer embryos at a time. The *NEJM* editorial pointed out that the United Kingdom regulates IVF clinics, with a three-embryo limit. When you plant three, they found 27 percent of the births will be twins and 6 percent are triplets or more. When only two embryos are implanted, the twin rate stays about the same, but there are virtually no triplets. Fetal malformations and deaths are significantly fewer.

If U.S. clinics agreed on a two-embryo standard, they'd be giving the fetus and the mother top priority, and putting the bottom line where it belongs, a little farther down. What a birthday present that would be for Louise Brown!

May Day

When they danced around the fertility pole in May, back in the fifteenth century, not everybody was enjoying it as a theoretical exercise. For childless couples, it was an occasion for fervent prayer, an anguished plea: Give us a baby. That sigh of pain hasn't changed much. In the U.S., one married couple out of every twelve really want a baby, and haven't been able to have one. Fertility drugs and embryo transplants are more effective than the May pole dance, but also more costly and dangerous.

Follow us through the story of the twentieth century worship of fertility, and see why: The demand for fertility treatment increased 300 percent in the fourteen years between 1968 and 1982. The reason was technology that worked. Promoted by highly profitable clinics in a competitive market, the new procedures have given hope to thousands of couples. But it's not like the old days, when every citizen could take a turn around the May pole. The Project HOPE Center for Health Affairs found that in 1992 it cost $67,000 for a couple who hit it lucky after just one fertility cycle. Those who needed six cycles paid an average $114,000. In tougher cases—a mother over forty years and an infertile father, for example—the average cost ranged from $60,00 for one cycle to $800,000 for six tries. These were only in-hospital costs, and didn't include the expenses at home after delivery. That's important, because of the dark secret of fertility treatment—the high cost of multiple births.

Fertility drugs can cause the prospective mother to release as many as ten eggs at once, rather than the normal single ovum. And, in laboratory fertilization, the clinic deliberately implants three to five fertilized eggs, in hopes they will succeed on the first try. As a result of these policies, in the seventeen years from 1973 to 1990, the births of twins rose 67 percent. The rate of triplets, quadruplets, and quints increased by 221 percent. The vast majority were the result of fertility treatment. Our instinct is to think of this as a cuddly statistic. But the reality is grim, even deadly. A *New England Journal of Medicine* article last year confirmed that when there is more than one baby, they are more likely to be premature, underweight, sickly, chronically ill, disabled, or still-born. After studying 13,200 births at a major hospital, the investigators reported that while only 15 percent of single babies needed intensive care, half the twins, and 75 percent of the triplets and quadruplets spent time in the ICU. And the more babies there were the more medical care the mother needed.

This leads to another, more troubling issue—what the fertility clinics call "selective reduction." Obstetrician/gynecologists are troubled by a rising number of patients referred to them by the fertility clinics. These are patients carrying four or more fetuses. The fertility doctors write a recommendation for "selective reduction" in hopes of avoiding the problems of multiple births. The idea is to leave two fetuses alive in the womb. It's a simple process; the doctor uses ultrasound to guide a needle through the abdomen, and a fatal chemical is injected into the heart of the fetus. Whichever fetuses are most easily reached are the ones to be "reduced." Why is this so troubling to people—myself included—who are pro-choice and accept abortions under certain circumstances? I think it's because these are intentionally created babies. They are the children of aggressive fertility treatment, by doctors who know full well that the use of multiple ova is likely to produce multiple—and thus endangered—fetuses. The hospital doctors are also unhappy that a life-or-death dilemma created by other doctors is passed on to them for resolution.

Will anything be done about this? Probably not. I have raised the question repeatedly over the last twenty years, without response. The ethics committee of the fertility clinics' professional association says it discourages the procedures leading to multiple births. But it has no teeth, and money usually will trump an ethical principle.

P.S.: Ironically, the "right-to-life" movement won't touch this issue. You don't read about fertility clinics being picketed or torched. These hard-liners are among those you might expect to be most critical of fertility treatment that inevitably ends in thousands of fetal deaths. Is it because they are at the same time so strongly pro-procreation that they help create the pressure for more babies, even from those who must agonize and struggle to produce?

Part Three	# Health Care

In Memory of Iqbal Masih

T ime for a reality check. A little perspective. Time to remember the people who care more about the patient than the profit. And especially about four gutsy groups of people who refuse to be seduced by the spirit of meanness abroad today. People who have learned from the turtle that you move ahead only when you stick your neck out. Your attention is called to a handful of ad executives, a big gaggle of doctors, five or six clothing retailers, and a twelve-year-old boy. The boy gave his life to make this a healthier place for other kids.

The doctors—They are the ones responding all over the country to the miserly and rapacious gutting of the welfare system. Forget the jokes about the golf clubs and the Mercedes automobiles; these docs are ready for civil disobedience on behalf of poor patients. They are especially outraged at the measure allowing states to cut off health care, including prenatal care, for children the politicians call "illegal immigrants." The doctors say they will not stop treating innocent kids just because somebody else broke the law in bringing them here. (By the way, a little perspective on this piece of legislative garbage: In the state capital where I live, there were 91,000 visits by poor people to county-run clinics last year. Only 639 of those were by undocumented aliens.)

The ad execs—They are a group of smaller New York ad agencies that are challenging the traditional ad-industry approach—the idea that they are not responsible for the products they're pushing. The group's name tells its startling purpose: The Initiative on Tobacco Marketing to

Children. They want it stopped. They don't buy their colleagues' claims that tobacco ads are not aimed at teenagers. They're now running ads of their own in trade publications read by other ad men and women. Arguing that children are "directly hit" by Joe Camel and his ilk, the ads ask media people: We can't close their eyes; can we open ours?

The retailers—Sometime before Kathy Gifford's widely publicized fifteen minutes of embarrassment an article I wrote described the sweatshops where women and children in near-slavery make expensive clothes for North Americans. It involved some of the most popular brands. Several retailers wrote or E-mailed to say, "If you can give us proof of this, we'll stop carrying those brands." The documentation went out, and it's safe to assume they kept their word, regardless of the pinch on profits.

Crusader against the sweatshops—Iqbal Masih came to the United States as a civil rights crusader, documenting the sweatshop story in a way ink on paper never could. Iqbal had been four years old when his family sold him to a carpet manufacturer. "For the next six years," says the English language magazine, *India Currents*, "he remained shackled to a carpet-weaving loom most of the time, tying tiny knots hour after hour." But when he was ten, the Bonded Labor Liberation Front helped him escape. He returned the favor by telling his story all over the world. A pint-sized, bright, engaging young man, he was the hit of the BLLF's 1995 international labor conference in Stockholm. He talked about terrible working conditions—children working from dawn to dusk in unsafe conditions, earning as little as three cents a day. "We had to get up at four and work twelve hours, chained to the looms," he said. Pakistan has six million child workers. Carpet manufacturers say their poverty-stricken country needs export dollars, and children's small fingers work best at tying the carpet knots.

As he traveled, tirelessly telling the story, Iqbal received death threats. He still owed the factory boss 13,000 rupees—about $420—of the money it had advanced to his father. The threats followed him even to Boston, where he received the Youth in Action award from a manufacturer of tennis shoes. The prize was $15,000, which he said he would use toward becoming a lawyer. He would attend Brandeis University, he said. Brandeis offered him a full scholarship when he was ready. "I'm not afraid of my old boss," he said. "Now he's afraid of me." But Iqbal was still a boy, and law school was a long way off. On a Sunday in April last year, he was with two friends, riding their bikes in their home village of Muridke, not far from Lahore. A shot rang out, and Iqbal fell over dead.

Some blame the "carpet mafia." If that's who it was, they acted too late. Thanks to Iqbal Masih's willingness to take risks, there are people all over the world determined not to forget the coworkers he left behind. Greed and self-preservation may typify us these days. If so, that will change. It will change the only way things always change: nudged ahead because somebody refused to settle for the status quo.

Double Effect

Nurses at a hospital I know were angry and confused. They demanded a meeting with their supervisors and the medical staff to ask: "Are doctors deliberately killing some of our patients?" At the meeting, one of them put it something like this: "Several terminally ill older patients have died suddenly after their doctors increased the order for pain medication. It looks as though it's deliberate."

"Nonsense," one of the others said, in effect. "That's always been one of the risks of treating serious pain. And people have a right to have their pain treated."

The reply: "Not if it kills them."

It was one of the livelier ethics discussions the hospital had seen, even if it wasn't new. People who care for—and about—patients have been debating it ever since the first painkillers were developed: How do you walk the narrow line between undertreated suffering, on one hand, and the lethal side effects of many analgesic drugs, on the other? Two things have added fuel to the argument. First, the movement toward doctor-assisted suicide gets its momentum from the very real fear that pain won't be adequately treated. This in turn is making doctors more sensitive to the way they handle pain. Second, all this discussion makes us aware that there are drugs, especially the barbiturates, that can kill, efficiently and painlessly. The states that permit capital punishment by injection use barbiturates, as do Dutch physicians legally assisting the suicide of dying patients. Barbiturates are recommended as reliable in Derek Humphrey's how-to classic, *Final Exit*.

So nurses' antennae are up when they get orders calling for these and other powerful painkillers. At the same time, these drugs are legitimate tools of the healing art. Doctors can order them and nurses can administer them without any intent of causing death. What they also know is that the drugs can weaken an already-feeble patient's ability to breathe.

Sometimes nothing else will help. The *New England Journal of Medicine* once told of a young woman with widespread cancer who signed over her decision-making power to her mother, "with the understanding that she desired pain control even if it could only be achieved at the cost of sedation"—keeping her permanently unconscious, with the risk of death. Doctors had already tried easing the pain and spasms by surgery, the maximum dose of radiation, intravenous anticonvulsants, muscle relaxants, and a spinal block. Eventually they granted her wish, sedating her with two powerful intravenous drugs and a facemask delivering nitrous oxide—the gas the dentist uses. Two days later she died of hypoxemia: not enough oxygen in her blood.

Did the doctors kill her? If so, can their actions be justified? Those are the questions that brought nurses together at lunchtime with a couple of members of the ethics committee, some cancer physicians, and nursing supervisors. Here are some of the issues that came up:

Most patients don't get the treatment they need for their pain. The American Society of Clinical Oncology (cancer) published a study of 1,177 physicians, 86 percent of whom said most cancer patients are undermedicated. The reasons? Well, these physicians put four at the top: poor assessment of the pain (mentioned by 69 percent), patients' reluctance to admit they were in pain (49 percent), patients' aversion to taking pain medicine (49 percent), and physicians' reluctance to give pain medicine (46 percent). The goal of pain treatment is too often tied to a specific amount of drug—not to relief. This may seem obvious, but many patients still go through agony the last two hours of a four-hour pain cycle. Part of this is the untenable argument that a patient could get addicted if the dose were increased. Philosopher-physician Eric

Cassell makes it sound simple: "The proper dose of analgesic is that which relieves pain."

Intent. The idea of double effect lets many practitioners live with the dilemma. That is, if they intend only to relieve pain, and not cause death, the second effect—the often foreseeable death—can be ethically justified.

Add a third effect: At a time when they're most vulnerable, patients' dignity and humanity are affirmed when we follow their wishes— whether we agree or not.

Unnecessary Pain

If you've been a patient in pain, the old joke may have a new punch line:

Q: "Does it hurt a lot?"
A: "Only when the doctor laughs."

A new government report raises again a puzzling question: How long will it be before doctors take their patients' pain seriously? How many studies do we have to have? How many horror stories? The new study indicated that half of all the people who have surgery are forced to suffer more than necessary. Why? Because physicians are reluctant to give them enough medication to ease the pain. The study was announced by Health and Human Services Secretary Louis Sullivan. A panel of experts did the work, going through years of studies. When they were done, they recommended new, more relaxed medical guidelines for patients in pain.

We like to think of doctors as cool, objective, rational thinkers whose acts are determined by scientific data. But, the fact is, they are human beings like the rest of us, and nothing proves it more effectively than their attitudes toward pain. Their feelings about pain, like ours, are more likely to be the result of religion than rationality. The Puritans may play a bigger role in their attitudes than pure science. Doctors aren't consciously cruel people. When they deliberately don't give enough pain medicine to a patient moaning in misery, they think it's because a real painkilling dose might make the patient an addict. When they severely limit someone's pain-relief medicine, they think it's because too much of it might kill a weakened patient. When they casually ignore the cries of a suffering patient, it's because they think of pain as a useful symptom, not as a tearing, wrenching agony.

They're partly right. These things are often true.

But more often the studies say, the physicians' subconscious is silently saying:

"Grit your teeth and bear it like a man."

"Pain can be useful as a warning; stop whining and be grateful."

"Appreciate the gift of pain; it builds character."

These are value judgments; they are based not on science but on a particular perspective on life. Many religions believe that suffering can lead to growth—but that's a long way from deliberately inflicting suffering to make the patient grow.

Helen Neal wrote in her book, *The Politics of Pain*, that "what we may think is an automatic response to pain and suffering most likely has been conditioned in us by the religious beliefs of our ancestors." This is why, several years ago, twelve prominent doctors from all parts of the country wrote in the *AMA Journal*: "People fear that needless suffering will be allowed to occur. . . . To a large extent, we believe such fears are justified."

This is why surgery still is performed on tiny babies without anesthesia in some hospitals. The excuse is that newborn babies don't feel the pain. But a *New England Journal of Medicine* article in 1987 is only one of many that refute this old idea: "In newborns, physiologic responses to painful stimuli are well documented"—and suggest that the trauma is "retained in memory long enough to modify subsequent behavior patterns."

This emotional baggage is why Drug Enforcement Agency officials have fought against the carefully controlled medical use of marijuana and heroin. Marijuana is the best agent there is for nausea in cancer and AIDS; heroin is a better painkiller than morphine, which is better—according to one recent study—than Demerol. The head of the U.S. Public Health Service injected another shot of reality at the news conference: Used after surgery to fight pain, morphine is addictive in only four of every ten thousand patients. On the other hand, Secretary Sullivan told the press, refusing to control a patient's pain can actually delay recovery. As the twelve physicians from across the country wrote in *JAMA*: "Under no circumstances should medication be rationed, because 'to allow a patient to experience unbearable pain or suffering is unethical medical practice.' "

The Widening Circle of Grief

The young man had been in the burn unit for weeks, fighting a battle all the nurses knew he had to lose. Burned over 90 percent of his body, he bore the painful treatments without complaining. The doctors spoke of his courage as something special, and the nurses would sometimes call in on their days off, to find out how he was doing. And when he died one bleak midnight, one of the nurses began to cry. The family doctor, who happened to be there with another patient, was livid with anger.

"Leave us!" He told the sobbing nurse. "Don't come back until you can behave like a professional."

It's easy to forget, when we're flat on our backs and in pain, that health professionals suffer too. In our hope that doctors and nurses can work miracles, we forget that they're human beings. We forget how often they must say "good-bye." One reminder of this fact came from Sallie M. Herrle and Bunnie Robinson, nurse supervisors who wrote in *Nursing Management* about the "turmoil" in a cancer-ward staff when a popular patient died. Herrle and Robinson say nurses who work with a lot of dying patients "are taught in school to give emotional support to patients and their families, but more often it is the nurse who needs support."

Patient G was a cooperative and genial patient with a devoted wife and two young children—"never demanding, always a pleasure to work with." As it became clear that Patient G was dying, the nurses' grief showed up in such symptoms as "irritability, argumentativeness, disinterest in the job and even . . . absenteeism." After G died, "the staff was an emotional turmoil for a long period of time. . . . Along with the relief [that his ordeal was over] came feelings of guilt and failure."

The turbulence eased, but only after a support group and counseling session gave them a chance to express their feelings of loss and anger, guilt and sadness. One of the hardest things, the group agreed, was the lack of a proper good-bye. "I went home after my shift," one nurse said, "and when I came in the next morning, he was gone. Somebody else was in his room."

Health-care professionals aren't taught how to deal with their own grieving—nor, usually, with others'. It has been a forbidden subject; stiff upper lip and all that. Ten years after she started medical school, Dr. Anne Peters wrote, "During those years I learned volumes of facts and information about disease and its many manifestations, but relatively little about an inexorable part of medicine—death." The cadaver on which she trained was impersonal, a lab specimen. She wrote in the *American Journal of Medicine* that it wasn't until her third year that she had to deal with dying patients. But she writes, "I never knew how to talk about death with the families, so I didn't." She felt uneasy about the sense of detachment she had from the patients who were dying, but didn't know what to do about it. "There was always another admission, or some pressing piece of 'scut' to do. . . . Then it all changed. My only sister, my dear friend, was dead. It was sudden and irrevocable." The first thing she had to do was track down her parents, vacationing in Europe, and break the news. "No training in the world could have prepared me to deal with the pain and disbelief in my father's voice. . . ." Two years later she was able to write, "I am no longer a stranger to grief. I know it all too well. But as I have healed, I have found that I am a better doctor than I ever could have been before. The feelings of grief and loss occur frequently in medicine—more often than I realized. Patients mourn the loss of a limb, the diagnosis of diabetes, the dissolution of a marriage, just as they grieve over the death of a loved one. Now I can truly mourn with these patients. Dealing with death is never easy, but I would like to think that future generations of physicians can learn about the feelings of grief without having to lose someone they love."

Dr. Malcolm Potts, a British doctor serving at the University of California School of Public Health in Berkeley, suffered that kind of loss, and wrote about the necessity of expressing our grief. He wrote in the medical journal, *The Lancet:* "My wife died in my arms, at home, three days after Christmas. . . . Grief is an astonishing emotion. It is the tally half of love, and it has to be."

If a doctor cries, or a nurse, he implies, it can be healthier for the patient's family—and for the caregiver—than bottling up the pain. Potts said that if he had been given the usual advice ("Take a Valium. Relax. Try and sleep.") "it would have trivialized my wife's memory and diminished me. Why does our society and our profession handle death so badly? Why are there thousands of love songs, decibels of rap, but not a single good hymn to grief?"

Nursing Home: An Eleven-Letter Word

It was hard to tell whether Jeanette L was suffering much. She had been semiconscious for several years—unable to speak or even nod her head in answer to the questions her sister Julie or the visiting nurse asked her. There was no sign that she knew what was going on around her, or even recognized Julie. She showed no reaction to a pinprick when a neurologist ran tests. Jeanette and Julie were widows in their seventies, and they had lived together since their husbands' early deaths, sharing duties, expenses, and a sense of humor. But strokes had taken Jeanette out of the conversation and then out of touch, and now she was slowly dying of Hodgkin's disease, a cancer of the lymph system. Exploratory surgery showed the cancer had spread; there was nothing to do but try to keep her comfortable. Julie chose to do that at home.

A home health nurse from Jeanette's health maintenance organization came by three times a week to check her condition and offer help. What she reported back to her department was not very pretty: Julie, the caregiver, wasn't strong enough to turn her sister as often as was needed to avoid bedsores. She tired easily, and often let Jeanette lie in her own wastes for hours.

These things made the large bedsore on Jeanette's tailbone almost impossible to heal. She would be brought into the ER every few weeks because the bedsore was infected again. Each time, Jeanette would be in the hospital for a couple of weeks, until the sore began to heal. Julie spent every day at the bedside. But when the doctor and nurses urged her to move her sister to a skilled nursing facility when she was discharged, Julie's answer was firm: "Not on her life. I'm taking care of her at home."

The home-health nurse disagreed. She brought the case to the hospital ethics committee.

Should she call the county agency for Adult Protective Services? Should she resign the case because she was just assisting and encouraging a situation that was getting worse, not better? "Why is Julie so insistent on keeping her at home or in the hospital?" somebody on the committee wanted to know.

"Well, she never came right out and said it. But I think when Jeanette first got sick, Julie promised her she would never put her in a nursing home. And she's keeping that promise, even though it's killing them both."

*   *   *

You've heard that promise, maybe even asked it, or given it. It has to be one of the most common contracts in the English language. It represents one of the gravest fears many of us have. That's probably a combination of factors, from bad experiences visiting in a poorly run nursing home to fears of being helpless, ill, and dependent on strangers for our basic needs. These fears aren't always justified, and the place you put your mother doesn't have to be like the worst one you've seen.

As a start, here are some clues to help you separate the decent places of long-term care from the places of quiet horror. They're based on advice from the Nursing Home Abuse and Neglect Information Center, reachable via Internet:

When checking out a place, visit it at different times of the day. Staffing is usually best in the mornings; the place may look much worse on a weekend afternoon—the time of lowest staffing.

Visit during meals, and find the assisted-eating dining room. Are the patients rushed, or are the aides patient and helpful?

Trust your nose. The rooms and halls should not smell like a toilet. Keeping patients clean is one of the main reasons a nursing home exists. Bedsores that aren't kept clean have a smell; clean bedsores don't.

Try to find at least one resident who will talk to you about the place. Don't rely on the guided tour, especially in the chain-operated, for-profit facilities.

Check out the bedridden or wheelchair-bound residents: Observe their skin quality, nail care, and grooming. Are their clothes clean? Is nearly everybody confused? Believe it or not, that's not normal for all the elderly. In a nursing home, a confused mental state can be endemic if drugs are used to keep the residents quiet, or if there is dehydration or malnutrition. Most states require a home to make available a copy of the most recent state inspection, or survey. If they balk at this, or at giving you access to the less-traveled halls, you may want to cross them off your list.

Ask an administrator how many registered nurses and how many certified nursing assistants (CFAs) are present on each of the shifts. There should be one CFA on the morning shift for each five to eight residents—more, if there's a high proportion of bedridden or wheelchair residents.

Our fear of nursing homes was highlighted when an eighty-five-year-old woman shot her daughter in the midst of a discussion about putting her in one. It doesn't have to be that way. The decent facilities and concerned staff are there, and finding them makes the extra effort in investigation well worthwhile.

The Spocks on Patients

There's more evidence that doctors aren't Vulcans, but humans like you and me. Disconcerting, in a time when heroes are in short supply. Unsettling to those of us who grew up on *Magnificent Obsession,* on Dr. Christian, and Dr. Kildare—physician-scientists who found out what was wrong with us by applying a piercing eye to a microscope. The news is tough, too, on the doctors themselves. From their first premed classes, most wear with pride the pointy ears of Mr. Spock—dispassionate, above the turmoil of emotion and bias, their distance and objectivity their strongest weapons in the fight against disease. That picture, like Dorian Gray's, has been getting really saggy in the jowls for a while now.

In the first place, medicine is moving in the direction of dealing with the whole person—the patient's mind, body, and spirit, in all his or her relationships, including the one with the doctor. Science isn't out of the picture, but it is seen in proportion to other factors, including the body's own ability to heal itself. Less focus on the magic bullet, more on the human being.

Second, we're finding that even in matters where scientific evidence is clear and relevant, doctors sometimes ignore it. What brings all this up is the news that most women with breast cancer still are advised to have mastectomies—despite long-term evidence that less radical measures work just as well. As the *New York Times* reported it:

"Researchers generally agree that women with small or moderate-sized breast tumors don't need to have the breast removed. The long-term outcome is just as good with surgery to remove only the lump, followed by radiation or chemotherapy.

"This conclusion is affirmed by seven studies, among thousands of women, with follow-ups as long as fifteen years. The National Cancer Institute affirms lumpectomy for women with stage I and II breast cancer and a tumor less than 2 inches across. This includes the vast majority of breast cancer patients. Dr. Sidney Salmon of the Arizona Cancer Center is quoted as saying that removal of the breast is justified in 'fewer than 10%' of the cases. Nonetheless, the American Cancer Society reports that the rate of mastectomies ranges from nearly 80 percent in one southern region to 45 percent in New England."

Why is this the case? For a decision so highly charged, so set about with social, ethical, and medical controversy, there's not going to be one simple answer. Those who counsel women with breast cancer say many of them equate eliminating the breast with eliminating the disease. The more that is cut away, the better. Others reportedly fear the side effects of radiation, such as nausea and hair loss, more than they fear loss of the breast.

That's their business. For too long, women were given no choice in the matter. Now that there are options, it's inappropriate to criticize the choices freely made by the person who's on the spot. A judgmental reaction is certainly improper. But it's that word "freely" that raises the question, and brings up the issue of doctors and scientific data. Dr. Marc Lippmann, director of the Vince Lombardi Cancer Center at Georgetown University, counsels hundreds of women. He says that when he gives them all the facts "most do not choose mastectomies." The problem, he told the *Times*, "is the doctors."

Researchers at the University of Colorado medical center have come to the same conclusion. They asked 175 breast-cancer surgeons whether they thought lumpectomies were as good as mastectomies, and whether they presented the two options to patients as equally safe and scientifically sound. Almost 25 percent said they thought mastectomies were better. Another 33 percent said the choices were equal but said they told patients that mastectomy was the more "standard" treatment. That's more than half whose patients may not really have a free, informed choice. When the information on which you base a decision is slanted, limited, or just plain wrong, the word "choice" doesn't mean much.

That's sad. One assumes these doctors wish the best for their patients, but what they're doing is ethically questionable. *The Times*, not known for doctor-bashing, says experts "speculate that doctors may have psychological difficulty letting go of the methods and philosophy of the treatment that they learned in medical school." And that "data alone may not be enough to force a change in medical practice, even when the statistics are unquestioned by medical experts." The good news is that the profession itself identified this problem and is working on it—moving toward a balance of objective science and kindly concern.

Both *Mister* Spock and *Doctor* Spock, so to speak.

Shifting Gears

For every dying patient, there comes a time when the doctors and nurses have to make a mental gear change. A time when they stop saying,

"Let's get the patient well," and begin to say, "Let's make this patient's last days as comfortable as possible." Obvious as it may seem, it's not easy to do.

Up until the last five years, a major problem in hospital medical ethics has been doctors' inability to make that switch. There are plenty of reasons, including physicians' perception that death is a professional failure, their own discomfort with death, and the fear of lawsuits if "everything" wasn't done. Hospitals have traditionally been places to "cure" people, not make them comfortable; it's only in the last few years, with the hospice movement and the rise of patients' rights, that many professionals have even been able to admit that they didn't have to keep on fighting for every patient to the bitter end.

Now that debate is winding down. (Although there are always a few who are slow to catch on; one week a doctor in one of the hospitals where I consult was told by a dying patient, "If my heart stops, don't resuscitate me." To which the doctor replied, "I'm going to pretend I didn't hear that.") In place of the old debate is a new question: Exactly what is "comfort care"? Is it withdrawing chemotherapy but continuing artificial nutrition? Is it stopping the antibiotics? Continuing the tests?

Consider this event in a hospital I know: A baby only a few days old was in the new-baby intensive care unit with severe, irreversible brain damage. After hearing the doctor's prediction that the baby couldn't survive very long, the mother and her family agreed that all-out treatment was inappropriate; only palliative care, comfort care, should be continued. Doctors and nurses agreed. But a day later the baby began shivering; even wrapped in blankets, she was chilling, and seemed very uncomfortable. A nurse put a tiny electric warming pad inside the blankets.

And the specialist in charge took it out. "She doesn't feel pain," he said, "Keeping her warm will only prolong her life."

The nurses grumbled, but had to go along. What was appropriate comfort care?

One problem is that the medical community has "professional standards of care" that spell out in detail the ways of helping people get well. But there is almost nothing in writing that describes palliative care. In recent months, a New York state task force called for standards, including:

Relieve the pain. Although this may seem obvious, many doctors are still not sure how much relief is "appropriate," and fuss on about such red herrings as "making an addict" of the dying patient, or weakening the body's resistance to death by giving as much medication as is needed. The task force said, "many health care professionals are reluctant to provide pain medication because they have an exaggerated sense of the risks of addiction and respiratory depression."

Recognize and treat depression. A competent patient's desire to end treatment is legitimate, but doctors are urged to be sure the patient is mentally well and competent. (It's now up to the doctor, by the way, to prove incompetence; the burden is no longer on the patient to prove competence.)

Be free to prescribe the most effective medications. This is morally acceptable, the task force said, even if there is a risk the patient will use it to commit suicide.

Some additional standards to consider:

Cut back on the testing. A 1984 article in the *New England Journal of Medicine* suggests that when a patient is "clearly in the terminal phase of an irreversible illness," much of the routine monitoring can be stopped. Yet, some doctors continue to order blood drawn, right up to the moment of death. The twelve authors said there is little point in taking pulse and blood pressure readings, X rays, and blood tests, unless they're aimed at some procedure for making the patient more comfortable.

Reassure the patient that he or she won't be abandoned. The patient is headed on the loneliest of journeys, and knows it. In this age of specialization, it can be a journey in which strangers are the only companions. Dr. Joanne Lynn, ethics chair of the American Geriatric Society, told a Senate hearing on reform that we should pay more for comfort care by the familiar family doctor than for a bevy of unfamiliar specialists.

Keep the communication open. Many doctors, nurses, and family members act as though there is a gag order on the subject of dying. Frank, open discussion—when it's clear the patient wants it—can end the cocoon of silence that surrounds many dying patients. For many dying people, this silence creates their most agonizing pain.

Part Four | DNA

The Double Helix

When Francis Harry Compton Crick and James D. Watson were carrying on the nonstop dialogue that led to discovery of the molecular structure of genes, they may well have given passing thought to the Nobel prize. But you can be sure of this: They did not expect their discovery to be used to authenticate rumors of extramarital affairs by two United States presidents who served 180 years apart. Nor did they foresee their discovery being used to catch murderers and rapists. Or, unscrambling babies switched in the maternity ward. Or, to identify the Unknown Airman in the most-honored tomb at Arlington Cemetery. Crick and Watson discovered the double helix—the shape of DNA—in 1953. Their Nobel came along nine years later. And it was 1998, forty-five years after the discovery, that the world really began to feel the effects.

Consider some examples:

The scientific journal *Nature* reported strong evidence that some descendants of Sally Hemmings, one of President Thomas Jefferson's slaves, are also descended from Jefferson. The genetic markers disproved the story, long told by some of Jefferson's heirs, that certain of Sally Hemmings's descendants looked like Jefferson only because the president's nephews had been intimate with her. Historians would have to rethink their assertions that the Jefferson-Hemmings relationship was friendly, not sexual. DNA stains on a dress in early 1998 appeared to confirm President Clinton's affair with an intern. Historian Joseph Ellis pointed out another coincidence: Jefferson, who was president from 1801 to 1809, indirectly denied having an affair with Hemmings.

The nation's law enforcement agencies took another step toward using DNA in a very practical way. The FBI opened a national DNA database, comparable to the long-standing national fingerprint file at FBI headquarters. The new facility ties together fifty databases, one compiled by each state. If you're worried about privacy, however, you may be on the side of those who see more risk than benefit in the new agency. At first it will include DNA samples of people convicted of crimes. But, the FBI is clearly intent on including ID samples of anybody and everybody. U.S. history contains more than one example of bureaucrats using knowledge to gain power over people. Sen. Joseph McCarthy, in some of the country's darkest and most dangerous days, showed that you didn't even have to have the data. If people believed your assertions that you had the goods on them, you wielded power.

Civil libertarians also point out that 25 percent of the Fortune 500 companies have admitted using DNA testing to weed out potential employees with a predisposition for certain genetic diseases. If big business gets hold of your gene profile, you could become permanently unemployable. During the 1970s, when there was widespread testing for sickle-cell anemia, and again during the HIV epidemic, industry has shown remarkable enterprise in getting hold of people's medical records—even when it's illegal. Great Britain has had such a database for years, and has managed so far to avoid the dangers of leaks in the system.

Despite the fiasco with the O. J. Simpson murder jury, most Americans believe that DNA research is reliable. According to CBS news, 68 percent of the population consider DNA evidence "very reliable." Others see it as "sometimes reliable" (23 percent), "somewhat unreliable" (94 percent) and "very unreliable" (3 percent). U.S. citizens' confidence in DNA testimony has been helped by the cases in which innocent people were acquitted. Most dramatic of these is the case of two little Chicago boys, seven and eight years old, were charged with rape and murder of an eleven-year-old Chicago girl. Police said, "We are certain we have the right individuals." But, after a hellish month, the boys were freed, and a suspect was in custody whose DNA matched semen on the girl's clothing. Most prominent of those cleared of murder was Dr. Sam Sheppard. Although convicted of murdering his wife, he died protesting his innocence—and DNA evidence has since shown the blood at the scene to be somebody else's. DNA helped the grandparents establish that two baby girls were switched in a Charlottesville, Virginia, hospital—and backed up their petition for joint grandparentship. Now comes another kind of custody case.

Impressed with the way DNA could identify descendants of both Thomas Jefferson and slave Sally Hemmings, Janet Allen of Peoria, Illinois, has sued to have DNA prove that she is a direct descendant of George Washington. It's a new role for science: giving reproducible authenticity to the phrase, "Father of his country."

DNA or Not DNA

DNA can not only tie a suspect to the [crime] scene; it can also prove there is no connection. It ain't, as the song says, necessarily so. It's true that many prisoners—including many on death row—have been cleared when genes in their blood failed to match fluids at the scene. But, for Roy Criner and others like him, the whole thing is a cruel joke. Criner, thirty-two, has spent a third of his life in prison for a crime he clearly didn't commit. His nightmare demonstrates that the acceleration of technology is no guarantee that the human brain will be able to keep pace. Among the factors that keep prisoners who have been cleared by DNA still in prison:

- The fact that in many states, the burden is on the prisoner to prove innocence. In other words: guilty until absolutely proved innocent. None of this "reasonable doubt" stuff.
- New federal laws passed in response to the bombing of the federal building in Oklahoma City. These make it much harder to appeal a conviction, even when new evidence clearly counters the "guilty" verdict. They require that an appeal be filed within a year—in some cases, six months. And, they allow little or no relief from the federal courts in cases where a state's social climate makes justice for convicted felons hard to come by.

- A recent British case that casts doubt on the crucial belief that each person's DNA is unlike any other's, and British officials said that a DNA test had appeared to connect a suspect to a burglary—but a burglary he couldn't possibly have committed. The chances of such a false match are one in 37 million. But it was a match, at least on the most common test, which compares six places along the DNA molecule. A second test, comparing 10 spots, showed a difference between the two samples. Chances of a match between two people in the more rigorous test were 1 in 1 billion. Among national DNA crime databases, it is the first known case of two specimens' having apparently identical DNA characteristics. Experts had believed that DNA profiles—each person's genetic map—were unique. Now, they're afraid that hundreds, if not thousands, of people found guilty through DNA evidence will want to appeal their convictions. They also expect skepticism, of the kind shown by O. J. Simpson's murder jury, to increase among jurors. "Those genes are too small to see with a microscope; how do we know it isn't just a government trick?"
- Refusal of some prosecutors, judges, and police to admit they made a mistake. An appeals attorney told *Frontline*, the public TV documentary program: "They worked hard for months to gather evidence against him, and the prosecutor stood up and told the jury what an inhuman monster the defendant was. Now, do you think they want to go back and say, 'We were wrong; he's an innocent human being after all.'"

In Roy Criner's case, there wasn't that much evidence to start with. The victim was sixteen-year-old Deanna Ogg, who was found in a woods in Montgomery County, Texas, beaten to death and apparently sexually assaulted. Criner, a logger, was convicted in 1990 on the testimony of three young coworkers who said he had bragged about picking up a hitchhiker and having sex with her in the woods. Their testimony conflicted as to the woman's age, hair color, and numerous other details. His boss says Criner couldn't have been away from work "long enough to cross the street," but the boss was never called as a defense witness. An unsophisticated ABO test of Criner's blood didn't rule him out as a suspect, but thousands of others in the county would also have matched. DNA technology, still new, was not tried. Criner continued to swear he was innocent, and when his family got permission to have a lab compare the DNA in his blood and in semen at the site, they paid for the test.

The lab said the semen was not Criner's. The county prosecutor asked the state forensics lab to run its own test. The results: The semen couldn't have been Criner's. That's it. End of story. The prosecutor told *Frontline*—which reported two other stories of prisoners cleared but still in prison—that if DNA testing had been available at the trial, Criner most likely would have been acquitted. He said he believed the tests were accurate, but meaningless. They didn't *prove* Criner not guilty. Thus, no new trial. The Texas Court of Criminal Appeals agreed, 6-3. Criner, meanwhile, has eighty-nine years to go on his ninety-nine-year sentence, and may have run out of appeals.

Chances of a federal trial are slim, and the governor of Texas, who might have pardoned Criner or commuted his sentence, was running for president on a get-tough-with-crime platform.

It was no time to embarrass law enforcement, or seem to be soft on prisoners—even innocent ones.

Who Benefits?

Ethical questions about cloning, researcher Jerry Hall said, "should be left to others." Not a scientist's concern, he seemed to say at the press conference announcing that his team had cloned human embryos.

Wrong.

Hall was asked about ethics because his team at George Washington University said that it had created carbon copies, genetically identical, of seventeen tiny embryos. The "Who, me?" approach to ethics is common among scientists, many of whom see ethics as a slightly flaky endeavor best practiced by people not bound by the strict code of hard science. These researchers feel that the "pure" in pure science leaves no room for any value judgments, any influences not anchored in provable fact. The provable fact, however, is this: Value judgments, the "shoulds" and the "oughts," are as important to science as to any other human activity. They determine what research scientists take on, and what gets funded. (An example is the report by a presidential commission that research in breast cancer, like that in women's heart problems, is held back by a serious lack of funding. Meanwhile, overhead, the government was spending tens of millions to find out why astronauts get airsick.)

Ethical values also influence the way scientists do their research, for better or worse. (Example of the latter: the top physician who admitted that he had provided illegal injections of an experimental drug for brain tumor patients, using them as guinea pigs without informed consent.)

The GWU team's work with cloning got more ink, though. Ever since the '70s, when it burst upon the public stage, cloning has been the Madonna of bioethics issues—flashy, intriguing, and highly controversial, but of debatable redeeming social value. The response to Hall's work resurrected the controversy. Among the outraged responses was a demand by a Vatican newspaper, perhaps in the spirit of Halloween, that U.S. laws "discourage those who, without scruples, venture into a tunnel of madness and want to write a horror story, humiliating and offending all humanity."

Hall defended the work in a press conference, calling it a useful way to help couples trying to have a child through *in vitro* fertilization. He said creating several embryos to implant, instead of just one, makes it more likely that at least one will implant and grow to term. After members of the team told the press they were interested only in the scientific details and would leave the ethics judgment to others, Hall then made an ethics pronouncement: There were no ethics dilemmas in his work because the embryos with which he worked were flawed and would have been doomed anyway within a few days.

Wrong again.

The issues still are numerous; here are just a few:

Are the embryos human beings? Many people believe, for religious or moral reasons, that they are. A sizable majority, still consider these tiny clusters of eight or sixteen cells as potential humans—worthy of respect and thus not proper material for frivolous manipulation.

Effects of the manipulation. Is there damage that won't show up for months, even years? Can we find out without putting a child-to-be in harm's way?

Research rationale. It's true that the odds for getting a "test-tube" baby are better when several embryos are placed in the womb. But shortage of ova or sperm is rarely the problem in IVF. If one ovum can be drawn from the ovary, so can several; that's been the practice for a decade. Did we not get the whole explanation, or are there reasons for this research that the team thought would be less acceptable to the public?

Is infertility a disease? We treat it as one—defined by cultural habits that go way back, before overpopulation became a problem. But, even if it is, what is the amount of money and medical resources we should spend on "curing" it?

Misuses of the technology. In a 1978 book, *In His Image*, a wealthy industrialist had a baby cloned from one of his own cells, to take over the empire when he died. It has been suggested that a couple could clone a new baby and freeze the twin-embryo, either to provide perfectly matched organs in case of need, or to "replace" the child if it died. Social scientists, limited now to a pair of twins, could have 20 or 100 full-grown subjects with identical heredity. The ethics problem with all these uses is that we would be exploiting human beings for our own benefit—not theirs.

There's enough of that already, without going high tech.

And Why Not?

Why not?

If we know how to clone human cells, why not do it?

It's pretty clear that as a nation, we're fascinated with cloning. It has been in the headlines since we learned about Dolly, the sheep who is her own mother's identical twin. But our fascination turns queasy when the subject is not sheep, but human beings. Look at the way we reacted when Dr. Richard Seed announced that he not only believed cloning a human was okay, but that if somebody would give him enough money, he would accomplish it within eighteen months. Disapproval flashed from every point of the compass, including the U.S. Senate, the White

House, and a battalion of editorial writers. Ted Koppel, who knows his audience, had him on "Nightline," and people were talking about him on every commuter bus.

The consensus: This man must be stopped.

If the good Dr. Seed's goal was to demonstrate that there is more heat than light in our objections to human cloning, he seems to have reached it. He might get equally high marks for success if his goal had been to document the public's vulnerability to showboat science. Seed, sixty-nine, uses lab mice in a small room at the University of Illinois at Chicago to study the immune system. He is not on the faculty, nor does he appear to have done gene research since the 1970s. In a field where even a few days' absence from the lab is considered a serious loss, he may not be as far ahead of his field as his press announcements might indicate. What's more, he told the press that he would use his cloning to help childless couples.

While this undoubtedly caught the attention of millions of couples struggling unsuccessfully to have children, it has a hollow ring to it. It is hard to imagine anything cloning could do for them that is not done more simply with *in vitro* fertilization or forms of genetic engineering. It is tempting to conclude that Dr. Seed is either naive, or believes we are.

Nonetheless, we're still stuck with the question: Why not? Let's ignore gut feelings for a moment, and try using the old bean. Are there rational arguments for banning the cloning of human cells, or at least severely restricting it? Here are some that might pass the test of common sense:

- It's premature. Dr. Mary Healey, former director of the National Institute of Health, reminded TV viewers that human research must be preceded by a careful series of experiments, beginning in the test tube, then in mice and rats, then in larger animals like the primates. It would be wrong to do human cloning, she said, because a sheep and a few cows and monkeys aren't enough to tell us what we need to know. If cloning human tissue is ever acceptable, it must be only after a long process with the lower animals. Meanwhile, we're just learning the procedures. The danger is high that we would produce human clones that were disabled or malformed.

- Short-circuiting the environment. Over billions of years, the species have developed as separate forms of life. Cloning can short-circuit these, creating a chimera—an animal descended from two species. We not only don't know what the outcome would be, but we don't know how to predict it. The world is often troubled by exotics—life-forms moved artificially to environments where they have no natural enemies. The eucalyptus trees of the Bay Area are an example—brought from Australia by a Methodist missionary. They have become a nuisance. Australia had to build the world's longest fence—5,000 miles—to keep English rabbits from destroying crops on the West Coast. The millions of rabbits descended from a few pair brought out by a homesick Brit. By bridging millions of years of evolution, cloning can create new exotics, with unforeseeable results. This could be dangerous in sheep, but it would be disastrous—and unconscionable—in humans.
- Individuality. Each child of God is unique—and what makes us human is that we know it. We are the animals to whom it *matters* that each of us is different. Any process that weakens our individuality—whether it is biological or social—weakens our sense of humanity, of being a unique child of God.

Greed at the steering wheel. The difference between a reasonable profit and "get everything you can" is a fine line. Business seems increasingly to go for the short-term success, the mandatory rise over the quarter before—often at the expense of the long-term good.

If human cloning moves ahead, its direction will come from the big pharmaceutical and genetic engineering firms. Wall Street has four newsletters just to help stock speculators track the genetic engineering companies. Among these are the companies that have funded cloning research. While none of their scientists speak openly of human cloning research, it is clear from their track record that they will produce whatever makes the biggest profit.

Are those the hands to guide such matters as health, environment, heredity, and personhood?

Part Five | Noteworthy Cases

Long Live the King?

W ho's the real heir to the throne of France? And, aside from a few romantics and possible relatives of Louis XVI, who could possibly care? Well, at the dawn of a new century of science, it turns out that two of the most advanced laboratories in the world are eager to get started on a solution to that question. They plan to use cutting-edge DNA techniques to try to find out what happened to the eight-year-old son of Marie Antoinette and Louis XVI. We might soon know who would be in line if the French suddenly decided to give up their experiment with democracy. Possibly more important, they'll be sharpening their skills and learning more about the limits and possibilities of the most promising area of science and medicine today. It's just the latest in a series of fascinating questions—some of them many thousands of years older—that genetic engineering is solving.

Historians agree on the beginning of the little prince's sad saga. He was arrested with his parents during the uprising that became the French revolution. Louis and his arrogant queen, Marie, died without mystery. During the revolution, death by guillotine was a public entertainment, and there were thousands of witnesses. Their son, meanwhile, was locked in the Temple prison in Paris. He became Louis XVII when his parents died, but he was a scared, sickly little boy. Much of the time he was alone, without medical care, light, or adequate food. Most history books say that he died there after a couple of years, probably of tuberculosis. His body was said to have been covered with sores from malnutrition.

But there's an alternate story—one favored by the 100 or so claimants to the throne in the two centuries since. They believe that faithful followers got the little king out of there, and left an impostor behind to die. At least a dozen people claim to be his descendants. And they think the heart of the boy who died in prison—removed at the autopsy—might reveal the truth. The French society that guards the royal legacy agreed to let DNA scientists examine a heart they have been keeping in a crypt outside Paris. Tiny slices of the heart will be examined independently by scientists in Belgium and in Germany. They'll analyze the chromosomes, and compare them with the chromosomes in a sample of Marie Antoinette's hair. The pattern of bands on the chromosomes should make it possible to say, with a very high degree of likelihood, whether the heart belonged to Marie's son, or to the hapless impostor. Whatever the verdict, it won't please everybody. The heart's origin has been questioned, and it hasn't been well preserved. The chain of evidence has been broken by robbery, carelessness, and even a riot.

But those who long for a king's return—or who just love a good story—will be ready to add a chapter to the sad little boy's tale. And genetic science will have taken on another unusual challenge, and advanced the state of the art.

Ever since James Watson and Francis Crick discovered the shape of the DNA molecule, unexpected uses for the knowledge have been popping up. For example, the tests that offered strong evidence that Thomas Jefferson had at least one son by his slave and companion, Sally Hemmings. In 1998, Catholic authorities asked for a test on the blood weeping from a plaque of the Virgin Mary in a Kansas woman's home. The lab found that the blood matched that of the woman herself. DNA is already so widely used in crime investigation that the FBI set up a computer to tie together fifty states' DNA databases. Criminals leave skin cells on everything they touch. Rapists' semen can be compared with a suspect's blood DNA. Saliva on a cigarette contains DNA evidence, even after it dries.

DNA cannot only tie a suspect to the scene, it can also prove there is no connection. In October 1998, the FBI opened a database to keep track of such evidence. Years after Dr. Sam Sheppard served a prison term for killing his wife, DNA indicated that he was not guilty, and that an anonymous intruder was the killer—as Sheppard had claimed all along. As the techniques get more sophisticated, ethical questions come along more frequently. In tracking down a criminal, is it right to ask everyone in a village to give blood samples for DNA analysis? When the data can be given only in percentages, how can a jury make a wise decision? Should employers be permitted to require DNA testing of prospective employees—in case the applicant has a predisposition for an expensive ailment?

We can be sure of one thing: The surprises of the new century will include some growing out of new uses for DNA matching. The sad story of little Louis XVII is a good start.

Every One

If ever there was a twelve-year-old with a right to be cynical about the world, it was a kid we'll call Charles. One day he was a member of that widely praised and envied institution, the middle-class family. His father had a steady job as a civilian clerk in a Navy office. Charles was doing well in school and had had his share of friends.

Then his father lost his job. Within days, Charles was pulled from school and sent to work in a shoe-polish factory to help support the family. It was a three-hour walk each way, and there were ten hours in a workday. Then his father was jailed. Something to do with being careless with money. Charles would later call it the most humiliating time of his life. He knew that people with an income look down on those who are hungry and destitute. He and his school friends had echoed their parents' shallow stereotypes for the poor—they're lazy, they lack ambition, they've offended God and are being punished.

Now Charles was on the other side. While his mother struggled to keep the family together, Charles spent his nonworking hours visiting his father and desperately trying to borrow money to get him out. He begged food to feed the family.

Eventually things turned around. His father inherited money and was freed. The family resumed their old life. Charles became in turn a clerk, a reporter, a writer of sketches, and a novelist. But he was not like many who escape from poverty. He never forgot what it was like to be poor. He never lost his anger over the blind smugness shown by the well off. At the same time, he never gave up hope that the scales would fall from their eyes. You can see how his memory haunts the books: Fagan and his loft full of homeless boys, for example, or Mr. Micawber in prison.

In 1843, some friends urged Charles Dickens to write a political pamphlet denouncing the apathy toward child labor and the poor condition of the schools. But, Charles said he would instead write "a sledge hammer that would come down with twenty times the force of a political pamphlet." His sledge hammer was *A Christmas Carol*. The story doesn't lose any of its charm if we read it with the eyes of the desperate, scared little Charles. But it does take on some relevance for the present.

Scrooge says, "I help support the prisons and the workhouses. They cost enough. And those who are badly off must go there." And, the smooth-faced mega-ditto sheep call the talk shows, whining that the poor are somehow robbing them! Congress and the president forge "welfare reform" based on jobs that don't exist.

Marley appears, swaddled in chains made of "cash boxes, keys, padlocks, ledgers, deeds" and the like.

Scrooge: "Why do you trouble me? Why do spirits walk the earth, and why do they come to me?"

Marley: "It is required of every man that the spirit within him should walk abroad among his fellow man, and travel far and wide. And if that spirit goes not forth in life, it is condemned to do so after death."

And we see the gap widening between rich and poor, at a faster rate than in any other developed nation in the world. We read about the billionaires who do not share because it would hinder their stride in the only race that still has any meaning for them—the race to be richer than others.

Marley: "[Our spirit] is doomed to wander this world—Woe is me!—and witness what it cannot share, but might have shared on earth and turned to happiness."

We feign helplessness while the number of people without health insurance grows to more than forty million. And, the CEO of a huge managed care cartel—since cashiered and facing indictment—accuses community hospitals of being "parasites" because they don't pay taxes—nor profits to him.

Scrooge: "You're fettered! Why?"

"I wear the chain I forged in life. I made it, link by link, and yard by yard. I made it of my own free will, and of my own free will I wore it."

And the spirit of the raggedy factory boy, young Charles Dickens, refuses to give up. It insists that we will see the pendulum swing back from meanness to a generosity for the common good. It insists that we will stop praying, "Bless me, and curse the rest." That we will instead join in the generosity of the little kid on crutches: "God bless us—*every one!*"

Take Me Home

"The disease progressed to a point where there was no more they could do," Nancy Tuckerman told the press. "They reached a point where she could either remain in the hospital or go home. She chose to go home." Jacqueline Onassis's choice was one that more people are making—and may signal that we've come full circle in our uneasy negotiations with death. In the first half of this century, most people died at home, with the family; and the children, and grandchildren were part of the passing of the generations. Death might be terrible or it might be peaceful, but it was a part of the family's life. Death often came from pneumonia, "the old folks' friend," for which there was no cure, and which brought a less painful end for many.

Then came the era of miracle medicine. In the booming years after World War II, two things helped determine where death took place: Thousands who would have died a few years before were being saved by antibiotics, intensive nursing care, spectacular new surgical techniques, and artificial life support. Even pneumonia was held at bay. As a people, we began to believe subconsciously that science would outsmart death; that the *Reader's Digest* would come out one day with a flap on its cover: "Found, A Cure for Death!" The place to find this miracle was the hospital.

Meanwhile, the more we denied the inevitability of death, the more we came to use the hospital as hiding place for those who did die. The

ICU, locked and shielded from all but a few, kept us from having to face the reality of death. Dr. Elisabeth Kübler-Ross, in the 1960s, was the one who opened our eyes to what was happening. It began when she wanted to interview a dying patient and found that, in a 600-bed hospital, not one doctor would admit having a patient who couldn't recover. The result was *On Death and Dying*, the book that showed us that many hospital patients died in utter isolation—curtained off from friends and family, in a cone of silence in which death was not to be mentioned.

But change was coming. Two widely publicized cases helped bring it about. A son of Aristotle Onassis, who would later marry Jacqueline Kennedy, suffered a severe brain injury in an auto accident. In an irreversible coma, the young man was kept breathing by the new artificial respirator. When it became clear that there was no hope for recovery, Onassis ordered withdrawal of the artificial support. The morality of the decision was widely debated. The second case was that of young Robert F. Kennedy, described more fully elsewhere in this book. The respirator (or, in the term used more commonly in hospitals, "ventilator"), was new to medicine. Many of the most progressive physicians didn't yet know how and when to use it—much less understand the ethical issues it raised.

Author Richard Goodwin recalls: "For a while doctors held out some hope. Then about 6:00 A.M. on June 5, his brother-in-law, Steve Smith, came out, and I could tell it was all over. It was just a question of when someone could get the courage to pull the plug." In the aftershock, the California Legislature passed the country's first "brain death" statute, and later provided for advance directives, the so-called living wills. Most states followed.

We were growing wiser, learning to choose our battles in the war on death. The hospice movement was making it okay to talk about death, even with the dying, and okay to die at home.

Hospitals were becoming more human. Families were allowed in the ICU; some medical and nursing schools began teaching that you can't stave off death everytime. The death rate, they learned, is eventually 100 percent.

When Jacqueline Kennedy Onassis's time came, society was ready, and so was she. Letting go was no longer an unusual decision. When her cancer was diagnosed, she made out an advance directive, limiting aggressive care. During her brief hospital stay, knowing that the cancer had reached her brain and liver, she refused the respirator—and antibiotics for the pneumonia that had come along. When the doctors told her the facts, she asked to be taken home. It was time to let go. When she died the next night, it was in a setting far different from the lonely 1960s ICU described by Kübler-Ross. As her nephew, Joe, Bobby's son, told the press: "A lot of members of the family have gathered to be with her. There's a lot of love in her room."

Death Further Defined

Nobody knows for sure how different the world might be today if Robert F. Kennedy hadn't been assassinated. But, there is one landmark in medical history that we do know is connected directly to the young senator's death more than thirty years ago. A bioethics dilemma stumped his doctors as they attended his death. The fallout from that frantic, puzzling time would eventually change the ER and the ICU; spawn decades of bioethics discussion over so-called "brain death," and lead the fifty states to change their laws defining death.

Senator Robert F. "Bobby" Kennedy had spent June 4, primary election day, campaigning in Los Angeles. Eight years earlier he had run his brother's successful campaign for president. Now he was covering the same ground, in a campaign seeking peace in Vietnam and justice for the sick and poor at home. Senator Kennedy won the California primary, accepting congratulations at a victory party in the Ambassador Hotel. He urged his followers "On to Chicago!" where he would now be the favorite at the convention. A few minutes after midnight, he and his wife Ethel left the ballroom through the kitchen. Surrounded by campaign workers and supporters, he was shaking hands with the kitchen employees when a young man stepped forward and emptied a .22 handgun point-blank at him. Two bullets went into his shoulder, within half an inch of each other. A third hit him just behind the right ear, stopping in the brain.

Five other people were wounded, but less seriously. The senator fell backward to the floor.

In the pandemonium, Dr. Stanley Abo was the first to answer a call for doctors. A campaign worker pushed him through the crowd into the kitchen, so hard his suit jacket was ripped off. Kennedy lay quietly, semiconscious. His chest barely moved. His pulse was strong, but very rapid. From time to time, he would groan softly, "Oh, Ethel."

The ambulance came at 12:28 A.M., setting off another bedlam. After Kennedy and his wife were inside, the ambulance had trouble getting away, because it was surrounded by a frantic, shouting mob. Several times, the ambulance's rear doors were pulled open by people trying to get inside. At Central Receiving Hospital, two miles away, the ER doctors examined Kennedy and agreed that surgery was necessary. They arranged for a surgeon and an operating room at Good Samaritan Hospital three blocks away.

At Good Sam, the doctors agreed Kennedy's chances of surviving were "extremely poor." But the odds might be improved by removing clots and foreign bodies—including the bullet.

Kennedy had stopped breathing, and was attached to a "heart-lung respirator machine," as the records call it. The operation, began at 3:10 A.M. It didn't help much. The records quote a physician as saying Kennedy's condition "could be described as terminal." The patient wasn't responding to loud sounds or painful stimuli. Brainwave tracings showed no activity. Last rites were performed, for the second time, and Mass was said in an adjoining room for six members of the family. And the heart went on beating, artificially fortified by the machine. Over the next twenty hours, the patient's vital signs grew weaker—while the doctors engaged in a worried discussion about what to do.

It was not a medical question. They knew they had done all they could, and that Bobby Kennedy would never wake up. They could turn off the respirator, after which Kennedy would surely stop breathing, and would clearly be dead. Or they could keep on assisting his heart and lungs, for days, maybe for months, without any hope that he would ever wake up. That's what they *could* do. What they didn't know was what they *ought* to do. For nearly a full day and night, the fourteen doctors—and as many more consultants—asked themselves these questions: Once you have put patients on the respirator, was it murder to take them off? California law said death had occurred when breathing and heartbeats come to a complete stop. But this patient had both breath and pulse, thanks to the respirator. Yet, he had no brain activity. While the doctors struggled with their dilemma, news broadcasts talked of Kennedy's "struggle for life."

In the end, the ravaged body settled the question by giving out. Even artificially propped up, the heart and lungs couldn't carry on. At 1:44 the morning of June 6, some twenty-five hours after the shots rang out and twenty-two hours after it became clear that Robert F. Kennedy was "terminally ill," he was pronounced dead. Soon after the ethics crisis in the operating room, California's attorney general asked for a law adding a third definition of when death has occurred: the total cessation of all brain activity. Over the next few years, the other states also added the new criteria to their laws. "Brain death" has long since become a part of our custom and language.

We won't know what his legacy as president might have been. But his death at least helped clear up one of those confusing questions the new medicine had forced upon us.

Aloha

After ninety years and forty books, author James Michener was ready to die. He told his doctor he didn't want any more hours on the kidney machine, and within a few days he was dead.

Did Michener commit suicide? After all those years of advocating a moral core for life, did he end up thumbing his nose at morality and the law? Did his doctor, by agreeing to stop the three-times-a-week treatments, break the law and the medical oath to "do no harm"? Many people thought he did, and no wonder. We've been through several years of intense discussion about physician-assisted suicide.

"Jack Kevorkian" is a household phrase. The voters of Oregon, two federal appeals courts, and many advocacy groups have been seeking a law letting physicians prescribe fatal drugs for certain dying patients. Meanwhile, the voters of Washington and California, many church groups, the right-to-life movement, and the American Medical Association have been opposing physician-assisted suicide (PAS).

But the fact is, James A. Michener's peaceful death had nothing to do with this debate.

Nearly everybody on both sides would agree that what he and his doctor did was not—repeat, *not*—assisted suicide. A look at what did happen might help clarify the difference between PAS and Michener's dramatic choice. At 90, Michener had had a full and fruitful life. His books had entertained millions of people. Recently he had told a friend, "As long as the old brain keeps functioning, I know the desire will always be there. I can hardly wait to get up in the morning to get back to work." But something changed in the last few weeks. Some don't mind the two or three eight-hour sessions each week in a recliner, reading, dozing, or watching TV while their blood runs out one tube and returns, cleansed, by another. But others get weary of the rising discomfort and diminishing energy between the end of one dialysis session and the beginning of the next. The diet is rigid, too, and not that tasty. No matter how he felt about it, Michener was in an artificial situation—kept from a natural death by the miracles of medical technology. Had this happened thirty years ago, he'd have been dead two weeks after his kidneys failed. The wonder of dialysis let him work and enjoy life, as long as life was sweet. When that was no longer the case, he decided to stop the medical intervention, and die naturally.

It made the news, but only because of his fame. Eighty percent of the people who die in hospitals today do so after making the same decision, or having it made for them if they're unconscious. For doctors, the question is this: At what point should we stop extending this life artificially, and use our energy to make the patient comfortable and pain-free instead? It's called allowing to die, or letting nature take its course. It is "withdrawing inappropriate treatment," "the right to refuse treatment," or "passive euthanasia." One thing it's not is suicide. And your doctor is not committing murder. All the medical societies and the Supreme Court have affirmed this. In September, 1991, for example, the medical journal, the *Annals of Internal Medicine*, spelled it out for its internist readers: "An adult patient, who has decision-making capacity and is appropriately informed, has the right to forgo all forms of medical therapy, including life-sustaining therapy." The authors emphasize that the withdrawal must be done "in a humane and compassionate manner," with as much painkiller as is needed for comfort. I regret to say that many doctors remain ignorant of this legal and moral requirement, or mistake "allowing to die naturally" for PAS. As a result, far too many dying patients suffer needlessly.

Back to the differences:

One is "allowing" to die, while the other is the act of speeding up the death. Refusing treatment is a response to the overuse of medical technology, PAS responds to painful, drawn-out dying processes that medicine can't—or won't—alleviate. Refusal of treatment is openly and routinely applied in hundreds of cases every day. PAS is also widespread, but only as a secret and illicit act. Refusal has been a legal right for decades. Whether PAS becomes legal in even one state could be decided in the next few weeks. The U.S. Supreme Court removed one barrier by refusing to hear challenges to the pro-PAS law passed by Oregon voters. A ballot measure that would repeal that pro-PAS law is the next obstacle for its supporters.

James Michener's dramatic decision, meanwhile, reminds us that we do have a choice when technology overwhelms us—and that one honorable and legal choice is just to say, "Sayonara."

Interleague Questions

Remember when Mickey Mantle was fighting for his life, after a controversial liver transplant and a diagnosis of cancer? Some folks are still talking about how swiftly Mickey rose to the top of the waiting list. It brought back memories of one of his homers, still rising when it hit the scoreboard. In fact, if you're a fan of the foolishness called politics, you may have noticed that Congress still gets into a bench-clearing brawl now and then over a question raised by Mickey's last days. *When there aren't enough livers to go around, what's the fairest way of deciding who gets the ones we have?*

The shortage is severe. Somewhere between 5,000 and 5,500 Americans received life-saving organ transplants in 1997. But another 4,000 or so died because no organ was available to them. Meanwhile, 8,000 to 11,000 people—victims of accidents or stroke, for example—

took healthy organs with them to the grave in that year. Why did these organs go unused? Several reasons, including:

- Twenty-seven percent of the families of possible donors were never asked.
- Of those who were asked, about half said "No."
- Time ran out on an unknown number of organs before a match could be found.
- The current system of searching for a match, gives priority to patients in the same region, then in the state, and finally elsewhere in the country. For somebody in the wrong county, it can be too late.

Dr. Donna Shalala, when she was U.S. health secretary, told a joint hearing of Senate and House subcommittees that she wanted the regions made much larger, moving toward one national list. "Where a patient lives and which transplant hospital a patient chooses . . . can determine whether you live or die." That was the system that found a donor organ for the colorful Yankee slugger. In his small Texas region, he would have been competing against an average of only one other person for a given organ. Another edge: Doctors hinted that the outlook after surgery was good. That fit the principle of triage, which divides casualties into three groups: those too sick to benefit, those who will improve without treatment, and those who will improve only if treated. The third group gets attention first. Later, doctors admitted their choice had been made before they found cancer had spread to Mickey's lungs. As a sixty-three-year-old with widespread cancer, he wouldn't have made anybody's triage lineup.

The flap on Capitol Hill that was stirred up by Dr. Shalala, went on for several years, proposing to give priority to the sickest, and to stress regions less. The new rule would offer an organ first to the sickest patient; offer it in a much wider area; turn over the job of getting relatives' consent to the experienced staffs of local organ procurement agencies; and require hospitals to report every death to the procurement agency. Pennsylvania's Legislature passed such a law a few years ago, and organ donations there are up 40 percent.

Sharply opposed to the change in priority is the United Network of Organ Sharing, a nonprofit agency that oversees organ distribution on behalf of HHS. Dr. Lawrence Hunsicker, president of UNOS, is afraid fewer people will get transplants, not more. He also predicted that favoring the sickest—rather than the patient most likely to benefit— would bring down survival rates, from 80 percent to 71 percent. Senator Bill Frist (R-Tenn.), a heart transplant surgeon himself, argued that organs now can be preserved much longer than when the regional system was set up. He wants a wider net cast. One factor didn't get much attention from the lawmakers: From the beginning, the emphasis in transplantation has been on "plantation." Surgical teams tend to have fiefdoms where they can both "harvest" and plant each organ. They know that you don't get famous—or become department chair or win prizes—by sending organs off for somebody else to implant. Like a sacrifice fly, that pays off only in faint praise. For thirty years, transplant centers have fought to see that organs in their fiefdom had a donor in their fiefdom. The bigger the center, the more would-be recipients it has—and the longer its reach for organs. Like the Yankees, the big ones have the payroll; like the Athletics, the rest might have to settle for moral victories.

How would Mickey have fared under the new rules? Well, regional distribution clearly helped him get an organ. That would change. After the truth about his condition came out, he was clearly the sickest guy around, and might profit from the new regulation. As it was, his life after transplant was measured in weeks. Before he died, he hinted that it might have been better to let nature take its course—and let some-body stronger have the second chance at life.

A Truce to Terror

A few hours ago, I stood at a window on the sixth floor of the Texas Book Depository in Dallas stunned by the banality, the ordinariness of the scene. Cars, bumper to bumper, edged toward the freeway entrance and home. Two women cast long shadows as they hurried for a bus. The scene was as familiar as Dan Rather's desk or the main street of Cecily,

Alaska. The stills on the museum walls from the Zapruder film weren't really necessary; they run inside all our heads, frame by frame. Part of the scenery of our day. Standing there beside the pile of book boxes that shielded the assassin, there was shock at how used to the whole story we've become. And how thoroughly we've become used to the monstrous idea of violence as a solution to problems.

In the same way that the jerky frames of film have numbed us to the horror in Dealey Plaza, the incessant flashes of violence elsewhere have made it ordinary.

We see the separate acts. We rage at the assassinations and feel the fear and anger on a dark street. We cheer for the international police actions and the midnight trips to the gas chamber. But we miss the connection. We miss the fact that violence feeds on violence, gives birth to violence, is inextricably a part of all other violence. There wasn't a lone gunman here on the sixth floor in Dallas. There were violent millions: Everyone who perpetrated, or even assented to, an act of violence as a way of making the world better. The despair that came in that spot, looking at the piled-up book cartons that formed a shield, was from the realization that we have met Oswald, and he is us.

Got a problem? Threaten, punch, stab, maul, or shoot it out of existence. Religious fanatics holed up in a compound? Don't waste any more time negotiating; go in with guns blazing. Disagree with a neighbor's choice on abortion? Make her walk the gauntlet; rough her up a little. Blow the place up or set it on fire. Oil supply in danger? No time for diplomacy; send in the boys. Bomb the place into a parking lot.

Can anybody calculate the cost—even just the health care cost—of believing that violence is a solution? Start with the inner-city emergency rooms, where surgeons have so much experience with assault-rifle wounds that Army doctors come to learn their techniques. Add in the costs—after years of French violence had failed—of trying to solve the problems of the Vietnamese people with guns, bombs, and defoliant. Include the suffering of at least a third of the street people, many of them mentally ill—all Veitnam vets. Add those civilians made hungry and sick by that war who are now hungry and sick on our shores. Try to calculate the pain. Through tears, I look at a picture of the funeral cortege down Pennsylvania Avenue, and try to imagine those whose loss was much closer and deeper in wars from Grenada to Iraq. From the sixth floor window you can see a shelter for battered women, a big one. Beaten by men who themselves were beaten as kids.

All of it's tied together.

Bobby tries to pick up where Jack left off? Just squeeze the trigger gently. Dr. King way too uppity? Get him in your sights. Lie in wait for John Lennon. Make a try for Gerald Ford, Ronald Reagan. Is General Noriega, now out of favor, still selling drugs? Go into Panama with high-tech weapons. Consider later whether the hundreds of civilian deaths were worth it. Does a drunken motorist lead police on an adrenaline-high-speed chase? Forget the control procedures they taught in police academy; knock him around a little before you take him in. Is a truck driver stranded in riot territory? Pound him to a pulp.

The gun, found later in a far corner of the sixth floor, cost $12.78. It was ordered through the mail from a whole page full of problem-solvers. The exhibits in the Book Depository reminds us that JFK sent the first advisors into Vietnam. But they also quote him as awaiting the day when "war appeals no longer as a rational alternative." And the thing he'll be remembered for, the exhibit suggests, is the Peace Corps. He is heard saying, "Let us call a truce to terror. Let us invoke the blessings of peace. Mankind must put an end to war."

Whether it's war between nations, ethnic groups, or just two human beings, that word has never seemed more pertinent, or more urgent.

Part Six | Futile Treatment

With Justice for All

As if just sleeping, the patient lies on his back, a plastic IV tube running into each arm from bottles suspended above him. A bigger tube pushes air through a hole in his throat, making his chest rise and fall slowly. His daughter stands at the bedside, as if on guard. Twenty feet away at the nurses' station, the patient's chart holds the orders the doctor has written. At the daughter's insistence, it's a full-court press, including artificial feeding and artificial support for breathing and blood pressure. It's a familiar scene, but this one is a little different. The patient is 103 years old. The daughter is 88. She knows her father won't ever regain consciousness. But he's alive, and she has told the doctors she will sue them if they stop any of the treatment that keeps his frail body pumping and slushing. The patient has been there for months, and could last for many more.

How much is enough? When is it no longer the practice of medicine on behalf of the patient, becoming emotional care for the relatives instead? Any experienced doctor or nurse knows that some treatment for some patients is futile. Doesn't do a bit of good. Doesn't make sense, much less justify the cost. But the professionals disagree about what "futile" means, and when it is morally acceptable to say, "enough." Even when there's agreement, it's not easy to tell a daughter that any further treatment for her dying father is useless—that keeping him comfortable is the only care that makes sense. So two things are happening in hospitals all across the country: Doctors are increasingly aware of the extent of futile care they prescribe, but when relatives object to the withdrawal of futile care, the doctors and the hospital back down. They agonize about it; they resent it. But, they do it.

They do it partly because there's no "community standard," no general agreement on what care is futile—a situation attractive to malpractice lawyers. Equally important, compassion—or avoidance of conflict—makes doctors reluctant to go against the wishes of the family. So the "treatment" goes on. A cure that is no cure. Physicians writing in the *New England Journal of Medicine* estimated a couple of years ago that there were somewhere between 10,000 and 25,000 such patients being maintained on artificial support at any given time. One city is trying to solve the problem by agreeing upon a community standard—by getting hospitals to agree on what treatment is clearly futile. The hospitals of Denver, Colorado, are working together to define which medical conditions call only for comfort care. If they can reach such a community standard and announce it publicly, then aggressive treatment won't be provided in those situations. *American Medical News* suggested, for example, that as a starter the Denver hospitals might agree not to call Code Blue for resuscitation of a failed heart for patients with these conditions:

- Confined to bed with cancer that has spread throughout the body
- Children with the fatal liver disease, Class C cirrhosis
- HIV-positive with two or more episodes of the pneumonia (pneumocystis carinii) that is typical of AIDS
- Dementia requiring nursing home care
- Coma lasting more than 48 hours
- Multiple organ failure with no improvement after three days of intensive care

There's general agreement among doctors about these conditions. But, even these can generate a rousing argument among the doctors, nurses, administrators, ethicists, lawyers, and insurers involved in the Denver discussions.

Some AIDS patients live on for months, maybe even years, after a second bout with pneumonia. Parents of children with liver failure have gone on TV to raise money for a transplant; our love of children over-whelms the knowledge that the new liver is likely to be destroyed by the same disease. The dementia on the list might well include Alzheimer's disease, surely one of the cruelest maladies. The spiral goes only one way: downward. But, many families and many doctors would insist that such a patient isn't dying, and that it would thus be immoral to with-hold aggressive treatment of any physical diseases the patient gets while in the nursing home.

The rest of us should be thinking about such lists. Reform in health care, in order to reach everybody, will have to cut off some of the use-less treatment we now provide. The line that is drawn will be moral only if applied the same for everybody—thus meeting the ethical require-ment for justice, for fair distribution of care. To make sure of that, we all need to be involved in the debate.

When Is Enough Enough?

If you insist on it, should your doctor be required to give you antibi-otics for a bad cold—even though it won't help the cold a bit? Doctors do it every day—some because it keeps the patient happy or gives the appearance of effective action, or may have a placebo effect. Some do it because patients' wishes get higher priority than they used to. But how far can we patients push, in asking for treatment that the doctor knows is useless? What happens when the stakes are life and death, instead of sniffles and a headache? That question is being debated—under the heading of "medical futility"—among doctors, nurses, patients, and ethicists all across the country. For example:

Doctors at a Chicago hospital refused a mother's request that they use a high-tech artificial lung on her five-year-old boy, whose lungs had been shattered when he fell out of a second-story window. They knew the treatment would extend the boy's life only another week or so, until other organs shut down. But, in Minneapolis, a judge told doctors they must continue artificial support, as long as her husband insisted on it, for an eighty-six-year-old woman who had been in a vegetative state and dependent on a respirator for more than a year. Anencephalic babies, born without most of their brain, usually get only comfort care; 90 percent die within a week. But one such baby has been kept alive for nearly two years, with intensive therapy ordered by a judge at her mother's insistence.

In Denver, meanwhile, the area's medical facilities are trying to agree on a definition of futile treatment, creating a "community standard" of care. They hope to establish a list of situations in which aggressive therapy won't be offered. An example would be a patient who suffers a heart attack on the street, and can't be revived before arrival at the emergency room. The chance of survival to a thinking, communicating quality of life in such cases is less than 1 percent. The Denver guidelines will probably say that the emergency room has no moral or legal obligation to try to resuscitate the patient. All this is being discussed as a question of "futility," but there are actually other moral questions behind that one. Here are a few:

How does cost fit into this picture? Many doctors have the uneasy feeling that this issue wouldn't be with us if there wasn't such a financial squeeze on medicine today. Some see a plot; others call it a by-product of companies' more stringent cost controls by insurers and the government. On the one hand, cost is and will always be an issue for medicine. The money has been limited for a long time. Our society needs to find fairer ways to allocate medical resources, ways that affect all people equally, but choose we must. That process might well mean ruling out certain procedures; as long as it was administered fairly, it could be morally acceptable. On the other hand, when it comes to an individual patient and physician, few would argue that money should be the basis of decision.

How does "quality of life" fit in? Must we go on treating indefinitely just because we know how? At one hospital where I'm a consultant, a comatose 103-year-old man is a "full code," at the insistence of his 88-year-old daughter. The resuscitation crash cart will go into action any time his heart stops. Some argue that without thought and communication, it's not really a quality life, and the best thing for the patient is to do nothing but keep him or her comfortable. Others say all life is sacred and must be supported to the max, even an existence that is only physical.

Should the odds be a factor? Medicine, like other sciences, must play the percentages. A 1 percent change is almost nil—unless, of course, you're the one in a hundred who pulls through. How long must the odds be to call an effort "futile"? Or, should we insist on that rarest of conditions, absolute certainty?

What are the responsibilities of medical professionals? Recently a six-year-old girl, with severe abdominal infections and then a brain-numbing stroke, underwent ten months of multiple surgeries, intravenous feeding, and respirator support. Her mother, informed repeatedly that death was inevitable, still insisted on all-out treatment. But, when the little girl finally died, doctors were asking: "Was this really the practice of medicine? Was this consistent with the goals of medicine? Was it appropriate care? And, "Is there ever a time when the physician's responsibility is to override the wishes of the next-of-kin?"

Which Way to Turn?

Melissa was an only child, a cheerful seven-year-old tomboy. She was a good kid, even if she didn't always get the family rules quite right. One of those times, she took a swim in the big pool in the backyard. She wasn't supposed to go in alone, but it was hot, and she knew her parents were right there in the house. We don't know just what happened, or how long she had stopped breathing when her mother found her unconscious in the water. The paramedics weren't far away, and they got there fast. They worked with the latest skills and tools of cardiopulmonary resuscitation. It seemed like an age, but was only a few minutes before Melissa began to breathe. Her parents hugged and cried.

She wasn't conscious when they loaded her into the ambulance, nor when they moved her into the emergency department of the nearest hospital. They connected her to a ventilator to help her breathe. Still she slept on. It was two long days before her eyes fluttered open. John and Martha were ecstatic. All too soon they realized that something was wrong. Melissa's eyes were open, but she wasn't seeing them. Her eyes darted back and forth but didn't seem to focus. She didn't say anything. For Martha and John R., her parents, it was the beginning of a time so cruel they never could have imagined it. Melissa's life had been given back to them, only to be snatched away again and dangled just out of reach. The neurologist gave it a name: PVS, for persistent vegetative state. He told them that unlike a true coma, which lasts only a short time, PVS could go on for years. Unlike those in the peaceful sleep of a coma, patients in PVS could wrench your heart with false signs of recovery. Their grunts and groans might seem like attempted speech. They seem to waken and to sleep. They seem to react to loud sounds or to pinpricks, but only to those yearning for some sign that they're coming back. Melissa was not coming back, the neurologist said. With her strong young body, she might live on for years this way. But the only way out of her condition was to die. He said that in the United States at any given time, there are 10,000 to 25,000 PVS patients. None has ever come back.

That was two years ago. Melissa is nearly nine now. She lies in a state institution; John and Mary didn't have the technology to care for her at home. She lies on her side, pulled into a fetal position by contractions in her joints. The miracles of modern medicine keep her alive. She has a breathing tube again, this time through a hole in her throat. Nutrients and liquids go by intravenous tubing, directly through her abdomen into her stomach. Other intravenous lines carry antibiotics for the infections common in a hospital, including pneumonia. It is standard procedure to suggest to relatives of a PVS patient that a no-code order be written—"Do not resuscitate" on her chart—so that if her heart stops, there wouldn't be any dramatic attempts to restart it.

Her parents refused the advice. Twice a day, John and Mary come to the hospital. They talk to Melissa, though she shows no sign of hearing. Together they go through a procedure. It is a program devised for children with certain neurological damage—children who are conscious, and for whom there is hope. It was not designed for Melissa. But Mary and John live on hope. As they bend her legs and straighten them again, Melissa screams. Twice a day, her screams fill the ward as her parents move her arms from her side to above her head, and back again. Nobody knows whether Melissa really feels the pain or not. But the cries are torture for the nurses on the ward. They ask, "In a case where there's no hope for recovery, must we let the family dictate aggressive treatment?

Or should we be keeping her as comfortable as possible?" They ask, "Does our responsibility for comfort care include stopping the parents from inflicting pain?" And, they ask, "If we tried to stop the parents, would the hospital back us up?"

The Unexpected

About 9:30 on a fall morning in the pediatric intensive care unit of a San Francisco hospital, a pediatrician injected a nine-year-old girl with an overdose of potassium chloride. Within minutes the youngster's heart stopped beating. Why would a doctor with sixteen years of loving service to children do such a thing? Look for the answer in legal documents of the state Medical Board, as they describe the last fifteen days of the patient's short life. Ask not only, "Why?" but, "What would I have done?"

The patient—let's call her Kim—had been suffering since birth with a nerve-and-muscle disease. She had come to the hospital for surgery on her jaw. After the surgery, Kim didn't regain strength. Days went by, and she couldn't breathe without help from a mechanical ventilator. After five days, the youngster's troubles took a terrible turn: When the ventilator tube was removed from her throat, she suffered cardiac arrest. Resuscitation took a long time, and lack of oxygen caused severe damage to the girl's brain. The next five days were crucial: Tests showed how serious the damage was, and Dr. C was rotated to the pediatric intensive care unit (PICU). Kim showed no signs of coming out of the coma. Finally, eleven days after the operation, Dr. C called together Kim's pediatrician, an anesthesiologist, and a pediatric neurologist. They agreed: There was no evidence that Kim would regain consciousness.

They talked with Kim's mother, who agreed to a "Do Not Resuscitate" order. If Kim's heart stopped again, nobody would try to revive her. Four days later the same four doctors met. It was a solemn gathering. The neurologist confirmed "profound, irreversible brain damage," and suggested that life support was no longer appropriate treatment. Kim's mother agreed, and the next day asked Dr. C to withdraw the ventilator.

About 4:00 P.M. Dr. C complied. As often happens, Kim went right on breathing, but raggedly, gasping for air. Although Kim showed no other sign that she could feel pain, Dr. C tried to ensure her comfort with regular doses of painkilling medicines—an opioid, Fentanyl; a central nervous system depressant, Versed; a barbiturate, Nembutal; and a relaxant, Valium. As the evening wore on, Kim became very pale; her lips turned blue. But the hard part was her breathing. Doctors call it "agonal" breathing, and it's no coincidence that the word "agony" comes from the same source. Even though she was comatose, and heavily sedated on top of that, the pattern of hoarse gasps gave the impression of a little girl suffering. In the words of the Medical Board's legal charge, Kim's mother became "more and more distraught" as the night dragged on. Finally, at 1:00 A.M., she asked the resident on duty to give Kim a large shot of "something" to end the suffering. The resident refused a deliberate life-ending act, but did step up the painkilling medications. She ordered morphine to be given as often as every fifteen minutes, at the request of either the nurse or Kim's mother. Still, rasping, gasping breathing filled the dim bay of the ICU. The next morning, before she could get her coat off, Dr. C was confronted by a nurse, pleading that she "do something" for Kim. The doctor found the girl "ashen, moribund, with agonal gasping." Kim's mother then said she "couldn't take [Kim's] suffering any more" and implored Dr. C to "please do something to end this." Dr. C stepped up the doses of Fentanyl and Versed. There was no change. Again the mother, weeping, standing beside the little girl who had suffered almost from the day of her birth, pled: "Isn't there anything you can do?"

Here is the place you might ask yourself, *"What would I have done, if I'd been the doctor?"*

*   *   *

P.S.: Dr. C said, "Well, I suppose we could use potassium." Almost before the sentence was finished, a nurse was filling a syringe with potassium chloride. It's a substance usually given to patients with dangerously low potassium levels, but a large, rapid dose can cause a heart attack. A few minutes after the injection, the little girl's heart stopped.

Dr. C, charged by the state with "gross negligence," waived her right to a hearing, and accepted a year's probation. She'll lose her license if she violates the terms: practice under a designated overseer; take a course in ethics; break no laws, file quarterly reports with the Medical Board, and be willing to be interviewed by the Board at random times; and pay the $4,000 cost of the investigation and the $1,200 cost of overseeing her.

Does He or Doesn't He?

American patients have the right to say "no" to medical procedures they don't want. But does "no" *always* mean "no"? Consider the case of Mr. M, thirty-nine, who arrived at the emergency room in an ambulance, siren wailing. The pain in his abdomen, it turned out, hadn't been caused by the chili he had for lunch, but by a burst appendix. He'd been toughing it out since the first twinges a few days ago, and had waited too long before calling the doctor. While he was being prepped to go to surgery, Dr. L, the anesthesiologist, stopped by; Mr. M asked her to "be sure to have my wife show you the paper I signed." The paper was his "Durable Power of Attorney for Health Care Decisions," designating his wife as the person with legal power to make choices if he should be unconscious. The form also included a box where he could spell out his wishes, and in it he had written, "No CPR, no respirator or other life support under any circumstances."

Mrs. M explained to the doctor that her husband had prostate cancer, of the kind that was already spreading. "So if his heart stops, or he stops breathing, that's it. He doesn't want things prolonged. I've told him I'd go along with his wishes." Dr. L agreed, out of respect for her patient's right to refuse treatment. She assured Mrs. M that her husband's wishes would be followed. Mrs. M left to pick up a son at school and bring him back to the hospital. Her husband was getting an IV tube with the first anesthetic, the one to make him drowsy. Only a few minutes later, as Mr. M on the gurney was being wheeled to the operating room, a nurse saw that his face was blotched; he was having serious trouble breathing, and didn't respond when she spoke to him. It was an allergic reaction, with the kind of swelling that could choke him. She stopped the IV, and called for Dr. L. Dr. L knew right away that she had more than one problem. Mr. M could die within minutes if the swelling continued. A breathing tube should be put down his throat immediately, and connected to a ventilator. She knew that if she did this, it would buy time to treat the allergic reaction. He would probably need to be on the ventilator only a few hours—at the most, a few days. But, she had promised to honor Mr. M's wish, echoed by his wife: "No respirator or other life support under any circumstances."

What should Dr. L have done? Did Mr. L's "no" really mean "no"?

*   *   *

The groups with whom I discuss this case usually split right down the middle. About half say Dr. L shouldn't put the patient on the ventilator. They argue that when he filled out his Durable Power of Attorney, he was thinking of his cancer, and the medical travail that might lie ahead. They say that when he wrote, "under no circumstances," he made his meaning clear. He would have been aware, they argue, that things can go wrong in a hospital. If he had wanted exceptions to his order, he would have spelled them out. The other half argue that Dr. L should put Mr. M on the ventilator, pronto. When he filled out the form, they say, an allergic reaction to anesthesia was the last thing on his mind. When in doubt, they argue, medicine should always err on the conservative side, the side of continuing life. Death cuts off any chance of changing one's mind. The "no" side comes back with the charge of paternalism. For too long, they argue, doctors believed they alone had the answers to ethical dilemmas in medicine—and the power to impose them on patients. It is time, they say, to take patients' knowledge about themselves seriously. The patient, they say, is the only person in the world who knows what an acceptable quality of life is for that patient. On the other hand, says the "yes" side, advance directives—Durable Powers of Attorney or so-called "living wills"—are written for a time when there is no hope for the patient. In many states, the "living will" is not a legal document until death is imminent. "No respirator" means, "I don't want to spend my last days on one of these," not "Don't use one of these to bring me back to my usual quality of life." Those who would have tried to bring Mr. M back argue that we don't know for sure what he would have wanted in the circumstances. What were his true intentions? The other side, those who would not fight the allergic reaction, say, "He said, 'under no circumstances.' "

| Part Seven | Health Care Reform |

Rationing Health Care

So, talk about rationing medicine makes you mad. Let me tell you about rationing. Let me tell you about mad. The supervisors of my county met the other day to wrestle with the "health care part of the county budget." A lot of programs would have to go. It was an open meeting, and people could speak in defense of the programs they depended on, or had founded, or worked at. As the paper told it the next day: "More than thirty people approached the speaker's podium . . . Some gave impressive statistics about the good their organizations have done in the community. They came up with strategies to scale down their operations. They promised they could make do, if only the cuts weren't too deep.

"Others spoke of their own lives, about the neighborhood clinic they walk to that is the only place they can see a doctor, of living with AIDS and knowing their children will become orphans." Some blustered, and some cried. Some of the supervisors cried, too.

This year the county will get less than a third of what it had for county health programs a few years ago—when everything cost less. Your county may not be as hard up as mine, but your elected officials are making the same tough decisions: How to spend the money when there isn't enough to go around.

One of the programs scheduled to be cut was the Legal Center for the Elderly and the Disabled. The previous year, in just part of its program, it had helped 3,600 low-income elderly people fight for their disability benefits or mental health care. Ron Javors, on the center's board, said the center was willing to drop all help to mentally ill people, if the county would continue the rest of the funding. If that wasn't enough, he said, they'd stop helping those who are losing their houses.

The Foster Grandparent program is scheduled for the ax, too. It pairs up retarded kids with low-income seniors, to the benefit of both. The long-range programs, the ounces of prevention, are getting the deepest cuts: vaccinations, family planning, well-baby clinics, and education against sexually transmitted diseases. So are the programs the poor depend on; dental service for homeless kids will be cut 20 percent. Three of the six county clinics will likely be shut down, and the others cut back to three or four days a week. There is money for only half the public health nurses we had last year.

Tell me about rationing.

Medical students' hard work and a month of smart politicking may have saved one of the clinics, a downtown center that served some six thousand poor and minority patients last year.

The students, who spend Saturdays volunteering at the clinic, spent much of June lobbying the supervisors, county staff, their own school officials and executives of a big health conglomerate—which came up with $175,000 to keep the clinic open four days a week for a year. There were smiles, hugs, and backslapping at the hearing the other day when the supervisors agreed to save the clinic.

We're used to this process. We don't think of it as rationing. But when somebody comes along with a more just and reasonable way of making the decisions—setting priorities and evaluating each part of the program—duck for cover, because the fur will fly. Look at what they're saying about Oregon's plan to get the most care for the dollar. Look at the multimillion-dollar campaign to bad-mouth Canada—which gets better treatment for more people by cutting waste.

Ration? Not in the good ole U. S. of A.!

Maybe in your county the process isn't so agonizing. Cuts don't have to be so deep. But, even then, there's rationing. Choices that save or lose lives are based on eloquent advocacy, good or bad publicity, the clout of the clients, or the goodwill of elected officials. To say nothing of employers who can't afford health benefits for their workers any longer, patients weeded out by long delays at understaffed public hospitals, or those cast out of the system by the unconscionable annual rises in costs.

Doesn't make you mad?

Okay. But, think about it, at least—the next time your temper rises at a reformer's suggestion that there must be a more reasonable and fair way to spend our health care money.

True Reform

The words "health care delivery" have wrestled their way into the language, but they still make me imagine a white delivery van, a driver in a billed cap, and "Health Care" stenciled on the sides. It's the same vocabulary that has us talking about reform in terms of who pays the tab and who arranges our trip to the hospital. That's a mistake. It's *what* gets delivered that makes all the difference.

Consider the sad case of Henry Jeffrey, ninety years old, blind, and indicted for murder. Jeffrey's wife, Helen, had Alzheimer's disease. He struggled to care for her as long as he could, and then he shot her to death.

The story is all too common: Exhaustion. Pain. Worry over high expenses. These are the causes of most medical suicides and most health-related mercy killings. And they are the worries that fuel the strong popular support for doctor-assisted suicide.

Jeffrey, in poor health himself, had hired an attorney to sell the house, help get Helen into a nursing home, and find him a facility where a ninety-year-old blind man could get the assistance he needed.

He was worn out. He knew Helen was likely to outlive him and he wondered who would care for her. And he knew the cost of two rentals of new quarters could soon eat up the equity from the house.

Exhaustion. Pain. Dwindling funds. The tragedy is that these burdens are not necessary. True health care reform could make them go away. Consider:

End of the rope. In the United States, it's the family that bears the burden of caring for a patient with Alzheimer's—early senility leading to demented behavior. Seventy-two percent of these caregivers are women. They may be responsible twenty-four hours a day, and may never get a day off. The size of their burden is shown in a study by the Philadelphia Geriatric Center: "The health of spouse caregivers is substantially poorer than that of older people in the general population." They had "more diabetes, arthritis, ulcers, and anemia" than others their age not caring for a sick spouse.

Another three-year study found that 46 percent of the spouses of Alzheimer's patients in one program had all the symptoms of clinical depression.

There is a good network of support groups for the relatives of Alzheimer's patients, but it reaches only a small percentage. Until our society gives in-home caregivers the kind of emotional and physical support other heroes get—Olympic competitors, for example—there will be people at the end of their rope, putting loved ones out of their misery.

The reign of pain. "If there is a single message in the recent attention to the topic of euthanasia," says an article on pain by the American Medical Association, "it's that patients fear one thing more than death—pain." While pain is not much of a factor in Alzheimer's, there is plenty of research evidence that patients' fear is justified in conditions such as cancer and arthritis.

Richard Blonsky, M.D., then president-elect of the American Academy of Pain Medicine told a reporter in 1991:

"I'd like to say that there's been a surge of interest in pain control, but that isn't the case."

One reason is the chilling effect of the "war on drugs." According to *Health* magazine, the idea of using nonaddictive morphine tablets for chronic pain "shocks doctors, worries narcotics agents, and frightens would-be patients."

But there's one place where pain control has suddenly become a major medical issue: Oregon. Medical schools and big medical centers report a flood of new training programs in pain management. They have all come about since the state's physician assisted suicide law was passed. Until doctors learn to look for pain and take it seriously in every patient, 60 to 65 percent of U.S. and Canadian residents will continue to tell pollsters they favor doctor assisted suicide.

How long will the money last? Medicare offers little in long-term care. First you spend down all your savings, then you can have a bed in a nursing home, such as it is. Many requests for assisted suicide and many cases of mercy killing come from people worried that they will use up their children's inheritance, in a long and costly process of dying.

As a people, we need to recognize that this care—like police and fire protection—is a utility, a public safety resource. As a people, we need to share the cost so every person has a pleasant, dignified last home. Lessening these three burdens is not simple. Nor will they go away with the calls for doctor assisted suicide completely. But (1) support for care-givers, (2) commonsense pain management, and (3) a universal health care system will drastically cut the need—and at the same time make us a more humane society.

That would be health reform worth working for.

Long-term Issues

When we think about reforming health care, most of us visualize intensive-care units, with their array of chrome and plastic gadgets. Not nursing homes. In fact, we avoid thinking about nursing homes as much as possible. Among our darkest fears, only a little less scary than a Stephen King villain, are (1) having to put a parent in a nursing home, or (2) being put there by our own kids. But, the American Association of Retired Persons and other groups are trying to get us to overcome our phobia and take a good look at long-term care. AARP is saying that Congress needs to include coverage for long-term care in any fair, humane health care system.

Besides the obvious issues of high cost and scarcity of private insurance, there are three dramatic reasons for covering long-term care:

- The requirement that we "spend down" our savings and income until we qualify—as paupers—for the only public program that will pay for more than a few months of long-term care.

- The fact that when care is given at home, most of the burden falls on wives and daughters, whose average age is fifty-seven. A third of these "informal caregivers" are over sixty-five themselves.
- The uneven quality of care in the 16,000 nursing homes, 32,000 state-licensed board-and-care homes, and as many as 100,000 unlicensed homes.

The need to bankrupt oneself in order to get necessary care results from the fact that Medicaid was designed as a welfare program for the poor only. It replaced the "poorhouse," which did the job from medieval days until the middle of this century. But, the need for long-term care isn't confined to the poor, or even to the elderly. Children with severe disabilities, people of any age with chronic illness, stroke, or paralyzing injuries can require long-term care. The help can range from living in "extended care facilities" to receiving services at home from nurses and therapists. No family member is more than a stroke or an accident away from needing long-term care.

But, being in a nursing home can cost you from $30,000 to $50,000 a year, and there aren't many middle-class families that can afford that. If you're single, you must pay your nursing home bill until you have only $2,000 left in savings or assets. Then you can get on Medicaid. If you have a pension or other income, most states will let you keep only $30 a month income. If you're married, your spouse can keep more of your assets and about $1,500 a month of your income. But, in seventeen of the states, a nursing home resident with an income of more than $1,302 a month is too rich to get Medicaid—although that's far less than the $2,500 a month the nursing home is likely to cost.

Much of the necessary long-term care can be given at home. But, professional care can cost from $50 to $200 a visit, and the average cost at an adult day-care center is $30 a day. So wives (23 percent), daughters (29 percent), and other women (20 percent) make up 72 percent of informal, unpaid caregivers. (Would Congress have acted faster if men were the ones bearing this burden?) A sobering statistic: The House Select Committee on Aging said in 1989 that, as the over-65 population swells, women can expect to spend more years caring for aging parents than they do caring for children. Not that men get off free; a 1992 poll found that a quarter of all men over fifty-five are caring for a disabled wife, parent, other relative or friend. Another disturbing figure from a government survey: nearly a third of the severely disabled people over sixty-five have no one at all to help them.

When reform comes, it must correct our long-time neglect of those who can't take care of themselves. Even more than the high-tech medical miracles, our long-term care system will send a signal: It will indicate whether or not we are a truly civilized people, willing to band together for the good of all.

Physician Shopping

Suddenly, there's a doctor shuffle. People used to think of the doctor-patient relationship as a marriage for life; now it seems to be heading fast toward the one-night stand—or, at most, the summer romance. The reasons are obvious. The effect on our health is not quite so clear.

The compulsion of firms to "downsize" is forcing people to change jobs—and, usually, health plans. Squeezed by the need to cut costs, health care plans are merging, going out of business, or dropping great clumps of doctors. Other doctors, in order to maintain their income, are forging new alliances or going to work for health-maintenance organizations. Which means a lot of us have to look for a new doctor—a process scarier than anything Halloween can dream up.

Time, then, for some tips on how to select a doctor you can, so to speak, live with. You've seen the usual lists; everybody from *Parents* magazine to *Money* magazine and *Nation's Business* has published such advice in the last few years. They include checking out the potential doc at the library—in the *AMA Directory* or the *Directory of Medical Specialists*—and asking the advice of pharmacists and nurses among your friends.

But the intangibles—including the doctor's ethics—are harder to psych out. Here are some things to look for in the first visit:

Watch out for burnout. For some practitioners, "Doctor is in" has been replaced by "Doctor is all in." These are tough times, emotionally and financially, for providers, and what began as a crusade can end up as life on a treadmill. Try to get a sense of whether your doc-to-be is just going through the motions, or still enjoys the challenge, the one-on-one dialogue, the curiosity that makes good diagnosticians.

Watch out for burnout (II). Chronic illness is no fun, and many physicians agree. They got into medicine to make people well, but soon realize that many of their patients won't ever get well—but won't die for a long time, either. The lift that comes with saving a life, or even drastically improving its quality, won't be there for many doctors when patients struggle with chronic illness. Try to find out whether the doctor you're interviewing has the patience for the long haul—or qualifies as bored-certified.

Tell me where it hurts. How does your would-be doctor feel about pain? No, seriously. Attitude toward the patient's pain may be the strongest indicator of how ethically sensitive a physician is. A doctor who takes pain seriously probably listens to patients and puts their needs first. Allowing patients to have a say about pain treatment is a sign the doctor takes patients' rights seriously. Studies show that physicians' practices in easing pain are influenced much more by religion and philosophy than by his or her medical training. Choose the doctor who cares how you feel about hurting.

Dying to know: How does your doctor feel about death? Studies show that on a scale of "fear of death," pre-med students rank higher than the average population. That's not necessarily all bad. But, some doctors never outgrow this dis-ease with death. Terminally ill patients make them uncomfortable, and while they may be sitting there across the desk from you, they have already subconsciously dropped the case. Some doctors refuse to face the statistics (the percent of us who will die is 100). They see each patient's death as professional failure, and either strive way beyond reason in a hopeless cause, or distance themselves from the embarrassing situation.

To tell the truth: The news that doctors have to tell us may not be so good. It may be very grim indeed. Try to find out whether the physician you're auditioning would level with you if the news were bad. You might be surprised to know how many docs there are who can't deliver bad news, and are likely to enter a conspiracy with your relatives to hide it from you.

So that's the "intangibles" list. If an apple a day hasn't worked, and life has handed you a lemon instead, your search for a new doctor can be a cause for worry. But the majority of physicians are men and women of integrity, well-trained and with your best interests at heart. The odds are on your side. Check out their rates and the kinds of insurance they'll accept. Find out their office hours and who will cover for them when they're away. Know what hospitals they have privileges in. And, then get the most important information: how they feel about truth, pain, patience, and death.

Poll Watching

One of those money-scattering foundations is looking into a system of government that just about everybody has considered at one time or another. Press a button and make Congress jump. The Americans Talk Issues Foundation reported a while ago that it was looking at the role of poll-taking in government. Well, actually, what it did was take a poll. Among other things, it concluded that Americans want to be polled before their representatives' decisions become final. Coincidentally, it was a week of polls on health-care reform—with results that demonstrated some of the problems of public polling as government. The American Medical Association, for example, released the results of its poll on reform. To the surprise of maybe a few, this poll found that Americans are wary of a government-run health care service. Not only that, but the AMA poll found that most people are willing—perhaps even eager—to pay more for health care if they have a choice of doctors and can get treatment when they need it.

The poll, by the Gallup organization, found that even more people felt that way than in the previous year. The results are a tribute to the power of advertising, if nothing else; the AMA, paid $1.6 million for a media blitz implying that government-financed programs don't allow a choice of doctors, and are rarely around when you need them. The results are even more impressive in view of the AMA's finding that the number of people with health insurance actually dropped 5 percent the previous year's poll.

Meanwhile, another set of doctors carved out a different constituency. The American Academy of Orthopaedic Surgeons announced that

Americans want health care reform, but don't want it too fast. The poll, released at the academy's annual meeting, concluded that 66 percent think changes are needed, but should be introduced slowly, starting with reforms in insurance, the law, and administrative waste. Those organizations can't have been too happy with the Louis Harris polling agency, which found that many more Canadians than Americans are happy with their country's system of health care. Although the AMA has spent the last several years reporting the miseries of the Canadian people under their single-payer form of government insurance, Harris found that the Canadian system is "more successful in providing access to needed services, engenders higher levels of consumer satisfaction with medical services, and is regarded much more favorably" by Canadians than the U.S. system is by Americans. Forty percent of Canadians and 14 percent of Americans said their system "works pretty well and only minor changes are necessary." The 40 percent, however, was a sharp drop from previous polls. Thirty percent of Americans said they would prefer the Canadian system.

Turning from North to West, poll-watchers learned that health-access groups in California had turned in petitions with more than a million signatures—enough to put a statewide Canadian-style health system on the November 1994 referendum ballot. Similar measures in Congress have the backing of ninety-six members and have been popular in several polls, but the administration doubts the votes are there for a single-payer system. As if in response to all this, Washington-watchers reported the AMA had increased the number of its lobbyists from six to eight, and the following agencies increased their spending; Planned Parenthood, the Christian Coalition, the AFL-CIO, a coalition of large insurance companies, Delta Dental Plans, and the American Hospital Association.

Somebody has a button that makes members of Congress jump, even if it isn't you and I.

Pop Quiz

The words "health care" are likely to pop up in conversation, no matter where you are. So is the unspoken question: *I wonder if they know what they're talking about?* So, here's a pop quiz, designed to help you bring a dose of reality to the table—and maybe a more solid basis for discussion—when the subject comes up.

Just put a "T" or an "F" next to each statement about U.S. health care, depending on whether you think it's true or false:

1. _____ Other than South Africa, the United States is the only developed country in the world that doesn't have some form of health insurance for all its people.

2. _____ About 15 percent of the population, or around 37 million people, have no health insurance.

3. _____ Most of these are unemployed or between jobs, including students, mothers with small children, and disabled people.

4. _____ When you get to be 65, Medicare will cover your nursing home care.

5. _____ Red tape makes the administrative expenses of Medicare and Medicaid three times as high as those of private health insurance companies.

6. _____ Thirty-two percent of Hispanics and 30 percent of African Americans lack health insurance.

7. _____ Although vaccination against the most common childhood diseases is widely recommended and is a cost-effective way of avoiding more expensive treatment, half a million children under the age of three go without it every year.

8. _____ Every year, 75,000 pregnant women go without prenatal care until the time they enter the delivery room.

9. _____ People can't choose their own doctor or hospital in Canada or Germany, where health-care spending is controlled by the government.

10. _____ Unless things change, the health insurance premiums that employers now pay are expected to increase sevenfold in the next few years—from an average of about $3,000 per worker to more than $22,000.

11. _____ High-tech procedures and other costly medical measures give us the best health care.

12. ____ U. S. medicine though expensive, has brought us greater life expectancy.
13. ____ Our system has at least brought us more doctors than, say, a national insurance system like Canada's.

Check your answers against these:

1. **True**. First proposed by Theodore Roosevelt in 1912, and resurrected by Presidents Wilson, Franklin Roosevelt, Truman, Johnson, and Nixon, full coverage has always run into roadblocks set up by those who had the most to gain under the old system.

2. **True**. In fact, in any given year, half the population is estimated to be without health insurance for at least part of the year.

3. **False**. Around 75 percent of the uninsured are working people and their families, employed in jobs that aren't covered.

4. **False**. Medicare doesn't cover nursing home care. Medicaid in most states will cover such care—but only after seniors have "spent down" their savings to the point where they meet the requirement: poverty.

5. **False**. Of each dollar paid to private insurance companies, anywhere from fourteen to twenty-four cents goes to administration—not to health care. Medicaid and Medicare take only three to five cents, leaving the rest for care.

6. **True**. Members of minority groups fall disproportionately through the gaps in the safety net.

7. **True**. Among the reasons: Cuts in federal funding for health education and preventive medicine, along with doubling and tripling of pharmaceutical firms' prices on vaccines.

8. **True**. Without health insurance, prenatal care is hard to find. State and federal funds for prenatal visits have been in a steady decline.

9. **False**. Citizens of both have free choice—unlike our uninsured, whose choices are severely limited. Under the most prominent proposals from the Administration and the Republican caucus, citizens would pay extra for freer choice of physicians.

10. **True**. A goal of all the proposed reform plans is to slow down the rapid rise in costs.

11. **False**. "Miracles" of high-tech medicine are certainly welcome, and put us ahead of other nations in such categories as saving

premature babies. But, students of our system are nearly unanimous in agreeing that our overemphasis on technology—at the expense of widely available preventive measures—is one reason we ran behind many other nations in such areas as infant mortality and heart disease.

12. **False**. U.S. health care, costing about $2,800 per person last year, appears to have no more influence on life expectancy than the systems of Canada, (about $1,900 a year per person), Germany ($1,700) and France ($1,650).

13. **False**. According to the *New England Journal of Medicine*, there are actually more doctors per patient in Canada. The difference in total cost for physicians' services is explained by fees that average three times as high, and by more emphasis on specialists: only a third of U.S. doctors are general practitioners; in Canada, it's more than one half.

Have a Heart

Are the drug manufacturers committing a moral wrong in their pricing of medicines for the elderly? Or is this just, as Walter Cronkite used to say, "the way it is." Are the big pharmaceutical companies squeezing us for everything they can get, or are they forced by economic reality to raise their prices three to five times as fast as inflation? This is a bioethics issue because for many Americans, the high cost is a matter of life and death—the difference between being well and being sick. This is especially true for the elderly, most of whom have no drug coverage under Medicare. Somebody has suggested that they are the only insured Americans without a prescription drug benefit. For such citizens, high prices can mean the drugs they need most are out of reach. In 1999, the price of the ten prescription medicines used most by senior citizens went up four times as fast as the cost of living. In fact, for five years in a row the prices of these drugs have risen much faster than inflation. For example, Schering's Imdur, for angina, went up 111 percent in the last five years. Just last year, it rose 9.5 percent—while the average costs of other medical services and products went up only 3.2 percent. Imdur's cost is $525 a year, by the way. Well worth it if you can afford it, or have a health plan that will pay for it.

The giant Glaxo is asking 88 percent more for Lanoxin, a heartbeat regulator, than it did in 1994. Glaxo and the other big pharmaceuticals assure us that, sadly, these price rises are absolutely necessary. Their reasons have the ring of logic: They say it can cost as much as $350 million to develop a new medication and shepherd it through the clinical trials required by the Food and Drug Administration. The drug must be priced high enough to pay for that, and for future research. For each product that makes it through the gauntlet to approval, many others fail. The cost of the failed research can come from only one place: the profits of the successful drugs. To sell the drug, they must spend money on advertising and marketing. The stockholders are entitled to a reasonable profit.

We're used to accepting these arguments without question, because we can see in their TV ads what warm, idealistic, and altruistic people they are. America has trusted the industry to set its own prices, and we assume they're responsible and self-policing. But let's examine these assumptions. *Consumer Reports*, Families USA, and ACT UP, among other agencies, help us out. The last has been blowing the whistle on the drug companies' impact on AIDS patients; the second spoke out for the elderly, as President Clinton tried to extend prescription coverage to them under Medicare.

These are some of the documented responses:

Research costs. The frequently cited $350 million figure was the upper extreme in an old industry study. Dr. Jamie Love, director of economic studies at the Center for the Study of Responsive Law, has said, "I know of no drug where as much as $100 million has been spent on clinical trials. The average cost is much lower." The Pharmaceutical Research and Manufacturing Association (the "Research" was added in recent years to add a little spin) reported in 1995 that the average research cost per medication was $24.5 million.

Failed drugs. The same study suggested an additional load of $30.3 million from the unrecovered costs of drug research that didn't pay off. Total research cost per drug: $54.8 million, or about $300 million short of the industry's usual figure.

Marketing costs. A Consumer's Union study three or four years ago stated flatly that it was the cost of advertising and marketing—not research—that drove prices up. The new tactic of promoting prescription drugs directly to the patient through TV—ask your physician about—has escalated the already high cost of advertising. Most prescription drugs are also impressed on the physician's mind by a personal visit from a "detail" man or woman. It's very expensive promotion, but it pays off.

Industry analyst Bob Roehr figures that in the budget for a new drug, 15 to 30 percent is for marketing and 20 percent for profit. That leaves "a lot of room for reducing drug prices and still not going bankrupt," he says.

Profits. What is a fair, reasonable profit?

Well, AT&T averages around 2 percent (net income/sales). Texaco and Chrysler average 3 percent. In comparison Glaxo—of the 88 percent price rise—averages around 23 percent. Merck averages 22 percent; Abbott, 16 percent; and Roche, 18 percent.

Pharmaceuticals, says Roehr, are "clearly the most profitable major industry sector in the economy."

Are such profits morally wrong? Are the prices that produce them an ethical disgrace? Does the heart have any place in daily commerce?

Except, that is, as the object of a two-dollar pill?

Part Eight | Issues in Mental Health

Still Dealing with Demons

What if the health insurance industry decided not to cover cancer anymore? Do you think there'd be an uproar? What if they dropped heart surgery? Can you spell outrage? Nonetheless, health insurers have maintained a long-running boycott on a collection of diseases that afflict twenty million to forty million Americans each year. Nine out of ten health insurance policies offer less coverage for this kind of disease than for the others. Yet, there's no massive protest.

Lumped all together, these maladies are known as mental illness. They're known for the suffering they can cause the patients and their families—made worse by unreasoning stigma and guilt. Although only a small percentage are dangerous to others, these patients are feared and shunned. Try to operate a halfway house for recovering patients, and you get the kind of neighborhood uproar that closed down one place in Berkeley a few years ago—leaving only twenty-three such beds in the whole city.

The outrageous truth is this: With health care available to more and younger patients, the number of youth and adults who "go postal" could be greatly reduced. To the family's emotional suffering, you can add the financial pain. Insurance companies justify their profits by spreading the cost across a large group, making care available to many who couldn't afford the whole bill. But they consistently oppose parity—equal coverage for either physical or mental ills—on the grounds that it would raise rates. The same could be said of any large-scale ailment.

117

How come it is taking so long to deal with this collection of maladies in a rational way? Why, at the beginning of the twenty-first century, is our response likely to be tinged with fear and superstition? A little later, we'll attempt a theory, but first, the good news. President Clinton has taken a step toward fixing the inequalities and lightening the unjust burden on the mentally ill and their families. With bipartisan encouragement from a score of members of Congress and celebrities ranging from Mike Wallace to Tipper Gore, he eased the path to parity. "It's high time our health plans treat all Americans equally," he told a White House health conference chaired by Tipper Gore, the vice-president's wife.

Immediate changes in federal regulations the delegates were told, will include these two:

- All 285 health plans used by federal employees must offer the same coverage for mental illness as for physical ones.
- Federal agencies must offer job opportunities to people with mental disabilities, just as they do for people with physical disabilities.

Because of the parity order, Clinton told the delegates, "Nine million Americans will have health insurance that provides the same copayments for mental health conditions as for any other health condition, the same access to specialists, the same coverage for medication, the same coverage for outpatient care."

Two members of Congress who have fought for years to get a parity law passed were present: Senators Paul Wellstone (D-Minn.) and Pete Domenici (R-N.M.). It was a sign that the Senate soon will hold hearings leading to introduction of a parity bill. Why all the foot-dragging? It's not just the insurers' obsession with profits. More likely, it's our unwillingness to give up myths that go way back before page one of the history books. Like our relegation of women to second-class status, or our bias against people of another race or sexual orientation, our fear of the mentally ill is a leftover from times when we really didn't understand what the score was. In the diggings of every ancient culture, archaeologists find indications that some people acted strangely—and that the blame was put on a demon. In biblical times, the treatment was exorcism. In various eras, the devil could be driven out by prayer, the drinking of a terrible-tasting potion, starving, or even flogging. Hippocrates, in the fifth century BCE. connected behavior to the brain, and unusual behavior to brain damage, but in the Middle Ages, religion took over again. Witchcraft—defined as dealing with the Devil—was the reason for abnormal behavior (defined any way the hierarchy chose). The punishment was torture and death.

There was a humane "insane asylum" in England as early as the thirteenth century. Seven hundred years later, bolstered by mood-altering drugs and new psychiatric techniques, we freed people from the mental hospitals, but failed miserably in providing the community programs that were supposed to take their place. We established health care insurance, but failed to include more than a few of the mentally ill. We say we blame the insurers, the public, and the politicians. Really, deep down, we're still blaming the demon.

Correction: We're blaming the afflicted person, for harboring the demon. That's why stigma and guilt are still part of mental health treatment.

The Pendulum

It was my parents' first visit to San Francisco, maybe fifteen years ago. We were walking down Market when we saw a man standing on a traffic island, brandishing a book and preaching at the top of his voice. He wore nothing but a well-used pair of brown oxfords. No socks, even. Later that day, my dad, who was seventy-five, was telling somebody else about what we'd seen. That's when I learned that it wasn't the orator's nakedness that Dad found remarkable. It was the fact that nobody was paying any attention to him.

Looking back, I realize it wasn't all that funny. It was too accurate a metaphor for the political plight of the mentally ill: the difficulty of getting anyone to pay attention. The network news was clucking worriedly about the Sydney flu, a brutal virus headed this way bearing nausea, fever, and related miseries. It is page one stuff, as it overcrowded the nation's emergency rooms.

Mental health isn't on the front page today, despite the fact that mental illness kills and disables more people than the flu—and all the other infectious and parasitic diseases together. Where is the news hour teaser about mental illness: "More people die and are disabled by mental illness than by cancer." As many as 80 percent of the people with severe mental illness are treatable, but the majority end up with chronic, often disabling symptoms—because in fact they aren't treated. President Clinton took a step toward fixing it when he ordered health insurers who do business with the government to provide mental health benefits on a par with the so-called physical ailments.

Some states, like California, consider legislation that will make it easier to commit mentally ill patients against their will. It's a tough ethics question. To some, it's a step back to the days when it was easy to deprive patients of their liberty. But, proponents argue that the pendulum swung too far. The bill, they say, would make everybody safer, including the patients. We'll see. In the 1950s and 1960s, well-intentioned legislatures freed the majority of people living in mental hospitals. If they were no danger to themselves and others, the idea was to treat them in environments as permissive as possible. As you well know, most states turned out the resident patients, but never arranged for the pharmaceuticals, therapy, and half-way houses so glowingly pictured in the original plans.

The rest of us made them invisible by not seeing them. They're like Patient J, thirty. J lives with his parents because the county ran out of money for the halfway house where he lived before. There they made sure he took his medicines for schizophrenia, and had the staff to handle him when he turned mean. J hadn't been taking his medications recently, and had spent three days in bed, fully clothed. When his sixty-eight-year-old father came in and stood beside the bed. J's booted foot shot out and caught him in the ribs, breaking two of them. "We love our son," his father says. "But I'm in no shape for that kind of thing. He was doing fine in a halfway house. When the county ran out of funds it was come back here or live on the street. It left just 23 halfway-house beds in this whole city of 150,000 people."

Elvira Gonzalez lost a daughter and two grandchildren to the weaknesses in our treatment for the mentally ill. For five years, Gonzalez had been trying to get her daughter into a treatment facility. But the laws now make it almost impossible to get help for the daughter, Julie Rodriguez. Gonzalez told a *Sacramento Bee* reporter that Julie's behavior had been increasingly erratic since a brother died in 1994. Julie invited her extended family for a Father's Day dinner, and just as people were sitting down, angrily dumped all the food in the garbage. She moved out on her husband, and accused him of tampering with her car. She said he was harboring strangers in the attic. She moved in with her mother, and then accused her of putting something in her food to make her angry. Her mother urged her to seek help,, but she refused. When Gonzalez talked to police, social workers, and county mental health workers, they said state law prevented them from hospitalizing Julie against her will. She had never threatened anyone, they said. She had a home, food, and clothing, so she wasn't gravely ill. Sometimes Julie would gather up her four-year-old son and two-year-old daughter and go for fast drives, with all the windows open, along the river. The mother called police each time this happened. "Something terrible is going to happen." But Julie seemed quite normal when interviewed by the police. Late in May, Julie took the children for one of her rides along the levee. Witnesses watched in horror as the car swung off the levee into the river. Police found no skid marks. Three days later they found the three bodies. The deaths were ruled murders and a suicide.

California is considering spending $350 million to make mental health treatment as available as the care for other illnesses. And, they probably will make commitment easier, but not too easy. That offers hope to thousands of very sick people—but probably little comfort to Elvira Gonzalez.

The Other Side of the Canyon

The road has been so long and bumpy, she says, that she and her husband sometimes refer to themselves as Thelma and Louise. But there's a difference: "We made it to the other side of the canyon." We'll call them Alice and Bill, and this is the story of their struggle with the ups and downs of bipolar disease—sometimes deep in a funk, and sometimes brimming with energy and wild good cheer. Alice is the one who needs "a mountain of strength not to take things that he says or does personally." She also has to deal with lack of understanding by the rest of us. "I'm outraged by the level of ignorance [about] mental illness." She points out that these illnesses "are more common than cancer, diabetes or heart disease and are the number one reason for hospital admissions nationwide." So, we find her in the pages of an issue of a mental health newsletter, supporting a controversial proposal that is gaining approval around the country: "I, for one, am a strong advocate in making certain that people with this illness—and other types of dementia—are required by law to take their medication." That statement raises hackles or garners nods, but leaves few people neutral. Here's their story; see what you think of the dilemmas it raises, of personal liberty, and public and personal safety:

Alice, forty-two, and Bill, thirty-four, have been married six years. Most of the anguish has come in the last three years—since Bill changed doctors and stopped taking his lithium. Bill's illness was diagnosed early in childhood. Years of treatment in his late teens and early twenties made him well enough to work as a missionary for his church, graduate with honors from a top university, and start a successful career in government. For ten years he took his medication faithfully. Then, a career move to the East Coast made it too expensive to go back to his doctors. Alice says the new doctor never sent for Bill's history or checked his lithium levels. "He took him off an anti-psychotic drug he had been on for over 10 years." Suddenly, three years into their marriage, Bill changed, entering a state of repressed anger. Later, he became manic; "his emotions just took off like a rocket."

Now that she has seen it many times, Alice describes what happens next: "There were terrible outbursts of temper where he would call me every horrible name under the sun. He would be totally unable to reason about anything. He ran up $30,000 in credit card debt in less than four months. He gave away material possessions, including his wedding ring, plus a replacement for it I had bought for him, and his prized college ring. He refused to take his medications, or be hospitalized. He would roam the streets, where on several occasions he placed himself in potentially life-threatening situations. He had a super-charged sex drive and sometimes exposed himself in front of our friends." He began to drink heavily. Life became a nightmare. Twice, after he attacked her, Alice tried to have him hospitalized. He behaved normally while the judge was present. Friends would ask, "Why doesn't he take his medications?" She could only say, "Because the neurons are cross-firing so rapidly, it renders the responsible part of the brain completely unable to recognize that anything is wrong." After such an episode, it can take months on medication "before it has really had a chance to kick in and start the healing." Many quit far too soon, and restart the cycle. In Bill's case, it takes nine months before he's well enough to comprehend that he must never stop the medications. That's why she argues for a new law.

The current law lets mental patients, even those who have been committed, refuse anti-psychotic drugs. The only exception: If a judge has found the patient completely incompetent.

"One would not think about letting a person with Alzheimer's roam the streets bereft of proper medical attention," Alice says. "Yet, people who are suffering from treatable mental illnesses are often neglected, placing themselves and others at risk on a daily basis."

Alice and Bill, after three years above the yawning canyon, think they've landed safely. Bill may soon be able to work again. But they worry about others, who never make it to safety.

Part Nine | Research

Voluntary Consent

When the kids were little, we played a game, "Mad Scientist," on long car trips. The warning cry, "Mad Scientist!"—upon seeing transmission towers, a silo, an overpass, or other landmark—meant that the car was under surveillance by that mythical archfiend, and everybody but the driver had to duck down below the windows to avoid his Death Ray. That warning cry has come back more than once, amid the revelations that Americans have been used as unwitting guinea pigs, again and again, by scientists. But, the scary thing is that the researchers who injected citizens with plutonium, without telling them, were not "mad" or depraved villains. Those who released radiation clouds on unsuspecting cities or ordered soldiers to take experimental doses of LSD were well-intentioned, with the best interests of the country at heart. Ordinary people like you and me. If somebody died—as somebody did when the Army sent flulike bacteria floating across San Francisco in 1950—it was seen as a regrettable but unavoidable casualty of the march toward truth (and, maybe, away from communism, the big bugaboo of those days).

Two things led these well-meaning researchers to the point where they could use such dismaying—and sometimes murderous—logic:

(1) Biological research requires intense concentration. The work takes on a life of its own. Real lives fade in importance, including those of families and subjects. It can block out every considera-

tion except proving the hypothesis; I've had more than one scientist tell me, in all earnestness, that ethics is irrelevant in the search for pure knowledge. Unfortunately, this naive conviction can blind the researcher to the realities of the research environment, ranging from the politics of grants to the mistreatment of human subjects.

(2) Ironically, it is a century-old ethical theory, to which many scientists unconsciously cling, that paves the way for subject-bashing research.

It's the utilitarian ethic, "the greatest good for the greatest number." The theory has had great appeal among scientists since the Victorian era; they can calculate and quantify the results of any choice, totaling up the effects just as Mendel could count his peas and the Curies their roentgens. It became the unquestioned assumption behind a century of experiments in which patients were kept in ignorance, lied to, harmfully injected, and mortally dosed. In its extreme, utilitarianism became "the end justifies the means." Never mind that some acts—like lying or cheating—are just plain wrong, even if their consequences might be a plus. But long after philosophers had come up with more realistic—and complex—ways of answering moral dilemmas, utilitarianism reigned in the "value-free" temples of science.

It wasn't that there was no guidance available from their peers. In 1949, the U.S.-led War Crimes Council issued the Nuremberg Code of human research, remembering the concentration-camp "experiments" of the Nazis. The first tenet of the Code:

"The voluntary consent of the human subject is absolutely essential."

According to a book by Professor Leonard A. Cole of Rutgers, in the next 20 years bacteria were released over 237 populated areas to find out how the bugs would spread in a germ war. People on the ground were never told. In 1964, U.S. scientists helped draft the World Medical Association's "Declaration of Helsinki," including this item:

"When obtaining informed consent for the research project the doctor should be particularly cautious if the subject is in a dependent relationship to him or her or may consent under duress."

Meanwhile, troops who "volunteered" were subjected to radiation and bacteria without the full knowledge of risk that is essential to informed consent. And prisoners in many U.S. prisons were able to earn cigarettes or time off by "volunteering" for medical experiments. The Declaration of Helsinki said: *"Biomedical research involving human subjects cannot legitimately be carried out unless the importance of the objective is in proportion to the inherent risk to the subject."*

Twenty-five years later, a doctor talked a mother into bringing her dying week-old baby back to the hospital so he could transplant a baboon's heart. It gave her seven more days of life, all of them filled with pain. It was only one of hundreds of experiments in which research was falsely presented as therapy. Human research is essential, and we all owe somthing to it. But, there is an idea in the Nuremberg Code that, if taken seriously by scientists, might have avoided much of the questionable research we've been reading about: *"No experiment should be conducted where there is an* a priori *reason to believe that death or disabling injury will occur; except, perhaps, in those experiments where the experimental physicians also serve as the subjects."*

The Ideal versus the Big Deal

The image of the scientist has been taking a beating lately. Those of us who grew up with mental pictures of selfless research heroes such as Marie Curie (Greer Garson in the movie), are taken aback to find some of today's scientists closer to the bumbling young Dr. Frankenstein, or maybe Son of Flubber. We see not only idealism, but also greed and ego. We see an anemic concern for the unforeseen consequences of their work. Take the announcement by researchers from New York University that they are working on still another way to get a baby for infertile couples. Dr. Jamie Grifo's team is using techniques similar to those used in cloning Dolly the sheep. Since some women over forty are infertile because their ova have deteriorated, the team inserted genes from a would-be mother into the hollowed-out egg of a younger woman. The egg is then implanted in the womb of the first woman, in hopes of producing a healthy child. In discussing the experiment, Grifo admitted that:

- No preliminary research had been done on animals. (Nearly all other biological research must be is done on animals before it is tried on humans, but the highly competitive—and profitable—fertility business has managed to stave off any government regulation.)
- Said they didn't do animal work because they couldn't afford it—since there are no federal funds for embryo work. (It's true that the religious right wing sets Congress's agenda on abortion issues, but "We can't afford it" is a puny reason for evading widely accepted scientific protocols.)
- Conceded that the research would have been illegal in states like California, which does regulate DNA research, and which is where he made the announcement.
- Argued against a cloning ban, saying it would harm his work, too. Grifo said the research had been approved by NYU's institutional review board, which must review all research on humans.

Another fertility physician whose acts raised questions recently was Dr. Russell Foulk. He was the doctor who "harvested" sperm from a nineteen year old man who lay dying from a gunshot wound. Jeremy Reno had found the loaded chamber in a game of Russian roulette. The request to withdraw the sperm and freeze it for later implantation in a surrogate mother came from the young man's mother, Pam Reno. Her reason: "I told them I have to get my son's sperm. It's the only way I can be a grandma."

Foulk admitted the situation required a closer examination before the sperm is used. "We're kind of in new ground here," he said. "We've not had the ability to do this until recently. . . . It's a request that is becoming more and more frequent." He added: "It's not different from taking organ transplants from a dying person." It is, of course. Organ transplants are for saving existing lives, not creating new ones. They don't raise questions about parenthood, possible birth defects, and the availability of such techniques to all. Reno said she would take a second mortgage on her home to pay for storage of the sperm.

Meanwhile, the three hundred or so fertility clinics across the country were abuzz with a medical journal's announcement that a new way of sorting sperm would soon let parents choose the sex of their babies with more accuracy. It raised the basic question of ethics: "Is this something we ought to do? On the way to an answer, we might ask: What is the purpose of having a child? Where's the pressure from to be a parent—or a grandma? What, if anything, will happen to the world's gender balance if we can choose our babies' sex? Whence the compulsion to have a baby that is "our own" (rather than, say, adopted)? None of these questions are meant to belittle the suffering of couples who struggle to have a child. Rather, the questions are directed at the fertility industry's commercial response to that suffering—an endeavor often apathetic about ethical issues and so expensive that many couples can't even consider applying.

Meanwhile, another gaggle of scientists was spending far more—some $3 billion—in a race that illuminates the ways science is torn between the ideal and the big deal. Government-funded labs in the effort to map every gene in the human body have been told to speed it up.

These labs, whose ongoing results are to be open to all, are racing to stay ahead of commercial labs—who are patenting every gene they find. The resultant monopoly on some of the new tests and cures will be a windfall for the profit-making labs. For a lesson in monopoly prices, see the pharmaceutical industry. Scientists are human, maybe more human that ever, and for some, the bottom line is fast replacing the common good.

Ethics and BWs

So, Saddam Hussein is playing hide-and-seek with his mustard gas and anthrax bacteria. And, a couple of guys are arrested near Las Vegas with what may or may not be anthrax bacteria *en route* to either fifteen minutes of fame or fifteen years in the slammer. It brings up a question that divided the medical community ten years ago. The right answer might mean—might have meant—longer life for you and me.

The question was this: Should doctors take part in medical research for the military? It wasn't a new debate. It was just heating up because we were haggling with the Soviet Union over on-site inspection—sound familiar?—and because of the new techniques in genetic engineering. We were able to recombine genes for health testing and therapy, but that also told us more about how to make people sick on purpose. As a result, the deadly calculations of mass destruction were beginning to be reported not in megatons, but in milligrams. For example:

Sarin—a chemical, not a biological agent—is the deadly nerve gas used by Japanese terrorists in their attack on the Tokyo subway in March 1995. Twelve people died and 5,500 were seriously hurt. Half a milligram of the colorless, odorless sarin is enough to kill an adult. It is twenty-six times more lethal than the cyanide gas used in some states' execution chambers.

But get this: Ten grams of anthrax, a biological agent, are more potent than a ton of sarin. Put it another way: A gram of anthrax bacteria is enough for 100 million lethal doses. Anthrax, caused by a spore-producing bacterium, is a disease found in plant-eating animals. You don't need a huge government lab to produce it, so terrorist groups (in addition to Saddam's bodyguards) will likely get it or make it someday. It's just one of many organisms, all of them more powerful than the chemical death agents. These biological weapons, or BW, were first used in war by the Japanese army in their rape of Nanking and the rest of China in the 1930s. Later, they did BW research on war prisoners, including U.S. and Canadian military personnel.

By the end of World War II, at least half a dozen countries had worked on large-scale plans for BW: the Soviet Union, the United States, the United Kingdom, France, Japan, and Canada. But, fear of mass reprisal kept the major powers from using their anthrax, plague, tularemia, staphylococcus, and Venezuelan equine encephalomyelitis. It wasn't until the early 1990s that Saddam Hussein's Iraq became the next government to use biological weapons, first in the war with Iran and then on rebellious Iraqi Kurds.

The debate that so divided the U.S. medical community had its beginning with a stunning gesture by President Richard Nixon in 1969. Nixon surprised the world by renouncing the use of biological weapons. He ordered U.S. stockpiles of anthrax and other medical killers destroyed, and he turned the germ warfare labs at Ft. Detrick, Maryland, over to cancer research. His gesture led to the Convention on the Prohibition of Biological and Toxin Weapons, negotiated by the U.N. and ratified by more than 100 countries.

The agreement had a loophole: "defensive research" was permitted. By the late-1980s, it was clear that the Pentagon was using the loophole to expand its biological research again. By now, Ft. Detrick was no longer a cancer center, but the Army's "Research Institute of Infectious Diseases." The Army insisted its mission was only to develop BW defenses. But, it argued, in order to stay ahead of the Soviets it had to know what new weapons it might have to defend against. The only way to do this was to research and invent new ones. And, of course this information had to be passed along to our allies for their defense. The principle of "no first strike" had become a "counteroffensive preemptive strike." That is, don't attack first, but if you think you're about to be attacked, you can attack first and really just be retaliating.

Meanwhile, some biologists were arguing that if we fell behind in this research, our nation would be fatally vulnerable to biological attack. (The Soviets still seemed a serious threat.) Others argued that it was ethically okay for doctors to do research on defensive measures like vaccines and protective gear, but not weapons of attack, like a stronger anthrax bacterium. Still others argued that war in any guise was immoral and that if medical science lent itself to agents of death, the arms race would come back to haunt us someday.

The debate never was settled, of course.

The dark side of medical research may really be our only shield from a terrible death. Or, its support from the medical community may have been what made it possible for that West German company to sell the ingredients to Saddam—so he could set up his own defensive research program.

Part Ten | Refusing Treatment

The Rest of the Story

Every physician in the country knows about the two Los Angeles doctors who got into serious trouble. And because they do, you may be paying a little more than necessary for medical care. Doctors Barber and Nejdl were charged with murder for agreeing to withdraw life support from a comatose patient and let him die. Chances are your own physician knows about those charges. Not the whole story, mind you—just the charges. As a result, he or she is likely to think "lawsuit" everytime somebody brings up the idea of withdrawing treatment for a dying patient. And, to practice "defensive" medicine, with extra tests and more procedures than necessary.

Most doctors in this enlightened day are aware of patients' right to refuse treatment. But, a hardy remnant still are reluctant to stop treating a dying patient, even when the patient pleads for release: "Not me. Those poor guys out in L.A. tried that, and ended up being charged with murder. . . ." Or: "I wish I could go along, but turning off the respirator would be murder." The sad part is this: Not one doctor in ten knows how the murder case actually came out. You can't exactly blame the doctors; the flood of information these days is far too much for a busy practitioner. It's hard enough to keep up with medicine, let alone the law. But folks, it's been more than a decade since Doctors Barber and Nejdl were charged. This is too long for costly misinformation to hang around. It's time, as the guy on the radio says, to get the rest of the story. Here it is:

Clarence Herbert, a patient of Barber and Nejdl at a Kaiser health maintenance organization, had undergone routine surgery. Shortly afterward, his heart stopped. The heart was restarted, but he remained unconscious, and he needed a ventilator to keep him breathing. Artificial feeding and liquids helped keep him alive. After several days it was clear to the doctors that Herbert wouldn't come out of the coma. Herbert's grieving family consented to have the respirator turned off.

But, like Karen Ann Quinlan in a more famous case, he went on breathing. The family was faced with the possibility that he might linger on in this state for years. Nine of them signed a letter to Doctors Barber and Nejdl, asking that all artificial support, including the artificial nutrition and hydration, be stopped. This, they said, is what Herbert would have wanted. The doctors agreed. Several days later, Herbert was dead. The family, whose beliefs included a life after death, were relieved. But a nurse who disagreed reported the incident, and it ended up in the prosecutor's office. For reasons that may have had more to do with politics than with medicine or ethics, Barber and Nejdl were charged with murder.

Now the big "secret." *The case was thrown out of three successive courts.*

When the prosecutor insisted on appealing, the California Second District Appellate Court gave it the final boot, ruling that:

- Physicians don't have a duty to give treatment that isn't effective. They may weigh the potential benefits of treatment against its burdens. Since artificial support would not return Herbert to conscious life, it was judged ineffective—and not a duty for the physicians.
- Criminal charges are inappropriate when useless treatment is withdrawn.
- The state does not always place biological life as the highest good, nor demand its preservation at all costs.
- When a patient can't communicate, it's appropriate for family members to give the consent for—or refusal of—treatment.
- Artificial feeding is a form of medical treatment, not a basic requirement of patient "comfort care."

In the years since, courts in many states have affirmed these concepts. Eight years after *Barber v. Superior Court,* the Supreme Court of the United States ruled that a patient's right to refuse treatment is nearly absolute, even for an unconscious person "speaking" through family members or other surrogates. And it ruled that artificial feeding is a medical procedure, not a cup of soup from Grandma.

But the misunderstanding of the California case rolls on. Its mythic power is stronger than the facts; its half-story is better known than the U.S. Supreme Court's conclusions. So, a case that actually freed physicians to respect the wishes of patients has ended up restricting many doctors to an overcautious, fear-filled approach to end-of-life medicine. There's another irony to this approach, the mistaken legacy of Barber-Nejdl: A physician today is actually more likely to get sued (or charged with battery) for ignoring a patient's wishes—not for respecting them.

The Key Question

The world may have stopped for Hugh Finn, but the governor of Virginia wasn't going to let him get off. You've read about Finn, the forty-four-year-old TV newsman who suffered a severe brain injury in a traffic accident. Since March 1995, he'd been unable to care for himself, feed himself, or communicate in any way. The doctors call it a persistent vegetative state (PVS), and there is only one way out of it: death. For Finn, high-tech medicine had postponed a natural death—pumping nutrients directly into the stomach for three-and-a-half years. He had been at two of the best rehab hospitals in the country for six months each and, finally, in a nursing home in Manassas, Virginia. Years earlier he had told his wife, Michele, that he would never want to live that way. She felt bound by that wish.

She told Hugh Finn's family that as his guardian, she planned to stop the artificial feeding. That set off a quiet but intense debate among the Finns—a large Irish Catholic family. It stopped being quiet after a younger brother, John Finn, filed suit to stop the withdrawal. Immediately the story was page one news, and reverberated from the Finns' home to the state capitol and the governor's mansion.

Why did it command such attention? Simple: It challenged one of the most strongly held beliefs by which we run our lives: The belief that we somehow are going to conquer death. This fiction has such a grip on us that we refuse to let the dying go. We refuse to see death as a natural part of life, and redefine it as an aberration, a cruel "act of God" like a tornado or an earthquake.

Look at what happened to Michele Finn.

- Hugh Finn's five brothers, his parents, and one of her two sisters all sided with John Finn in the suit.
- A sister who lived in Philadelphia alerted state officials and fed them questionable information about Hugh Finn's condition.
- Apparently as a result, cabinet-level state officials began publicly challenging the diagnosis of PVS—even though a state neurologist had confirmed the diagnosis.
- State legislator Robert G. Marshall led a highly publicized drive to keep the tube connected, as though these things were best settled by referendum, and organized protest rallies outside the nursing home. He announced that ending life support for Finn would be illegal and against the teaching of the Catholic Church. Neither statement is accurate.

Michele Finn, forced into public debate, told the press: "My husband is completely uncommunicative. He can't roll over in his bed. He has to have his diapers changed. . . . He has no quality of life."

County Judge Frank Hoss Jr. wasn't impressed by what he called the politics of the case. He ruled that pulling Huge Finn's tubes was neither euthanasia nor mercy killing, but allowing the natural processes of death to replace technology. He pointed out that ending artificial nutrition for a PVS patient was specifically permitted by Virginia law. When the Finn family decided not to appeal, Governor Jim Gilmore filed suit himself. There was a dramatic after-midnight hearing and an appeal to the state Supreme Court.

Political analyst Mark Rozell commented: "Gilmore is very much aware of his support among Christian conservatives. . . . There is not a huge constituency that would be motivated by sympathy for the family. But there is a very motivated constituency that is easily mobilized on the right. It's a no-lose situation [for the governor.]"

Freedom to Die: People, Politics and the Right-to-Die (St. Martin's Press, $24.95 in hardback) is the first book to tell us what's happening in a situation like the Finns'. It's the inside story of the forces that make up the right to die movement. Its coauthors are especially qualified. Derek Humphry helped found the Hemlock Society, and wrote *Final Exit*—a book that demonstrated, by riding the best-seller lists for eighteen weeks, how widespread the concern over freedom to die was. Mary Clement is an Arizona attorney and president of Gentle Closure, Inc., which "assists people in addressing end-of-life concerns." Although they have a clear point of view, the book is not shrill. Humphry and Clement keep it low-key and factual. Especially compelling is the first detailed discussion of how Oregon passed its physician-assisted suicide bill. The book is valuable as a reference, and for looking beneath the surface in the politics of dying.

As for Hugh Finn, the family came together for a weekend and asked themselves the key question in any bioethics discussion: What would the patient have wanted?

Not, "What do we think is best?"

"What would Hugh have wanted?"

The artificial feeding was stopped. The Supreme Court rebuffed the governor's last appeal. And, Hugh Finn got the freedom he had told his wife he would want in such a situation: the freedom to die.

The More, the Better

The surgeon was purple with frustration and anger.

"Twelve years I studied to know how to help that woman. Twenty years I practiced, mostly on cases much tougher than this. I know I can save her life with a simple procedure. And she won't give her consent."

He had just left the room of Mrs. M, a seventy-nine-year-old diabetic, whose infected toes were refusing to heal. Now gangrene was present in one foot, and seemed imminent in the other. Untreated, it would soon kill her. The only sensible course of action, the surgeon had told her, was amputation—far enough up each leg to stay ahead of the dying flesh. It was drastic, but it would save her life.

She said, "No thanks, doctor."

Now, an hour later, he was venting his frustration on an ethicist friend. "The woman doesn't even have a grade school education," he huffed. "Patients shouldn't be making important decisions like this."

There was a time—as he well knew—when patients didn't. Doctors were the decision makers.

As recently as thirty-five years ago, most doctors would have made not just the medical decision for Mrs. M.—*What is the best of all possible medical interventions here?* Doctors would have also decided the ethical question: *Would amputation be the option most compatible with her beliefs, values, and attitude toward life?* In those days, when a physician entered a room, the nurses stood. So did the patients, the ones who were able.

Change had already begun, but very slowly. For two hundred years, British and U.S. law had a tort called "battery"—roughly defined as touching a person without permission. You know, "assault and battery." The U.S. Supreme Court ruled as early as 1914 that doing surgery on an adult without permission was battery: "Every human being of adult years and sound mind has a right to determine what shall be done with his own body, and a surgeon who performs an operation without his patient's consent commits an assault for which he is liable in damages." U.S. medicine didn't pay a lot of attention. Awed by the growing scientific aura surrounding medical practice, most patients let the doctor decide, and the doctors were quite willing to accept the scepter. There was almost no discussion of "letting go," of stopping treatment when its burden outweighed any possible benefits.

That was partly because medicine, until World War II, was still a crude craft. Our doctors could use their most powerful weapons, as long as they could, and still not be in danger of overusing them. Patient consent began to make a comeback with the Nuremberg trials. Nazi doctors justified their fatal experiments on concentration camp inmates with the fact that the results might save thousands of (German) lives. That's why Rule 1 of the Nuremberg Code, which resulted from the trials, was this: "The voluntary consent of the human subject is absolutely essential."

Still doctors made most "should" or "shouldn't" decisions for patients. It was no coincidence that the late Robert Young could star in both *Marcus Welby M.D.* and *Father Knows Best*. But things were moving. All hell broke loose when Dr. Henry Beecher of Harvard published a medical journal article listing a couple of dozen medical studies in which patient consent had been ignored.

Then the parents of Karen Ann Quinlan, a young woman in deep coma, sued to let her be set free of the respirator that kept her alive. Devout Catholics, they had the backing of their bishop, but not of the doctors. In 1975 the New Jersey Supreme Court allowed the breathing tube's removal, and mandated the first ethics committees to look at future cases. Years later, the U.S. Supreme Court, in the case of another comatose young woman, would support the absolute right of patients to refuse unwanted medical treatment. If the patient was unconscious, the justices said, a surrogate who knew what the patient would have wanted could make the decision.

While all this went on, the world was "a-changing." Patients' rights were part of a movement that included civil rights, free speech, consumers' rights and, especially, women's rights. With a landmark book, *Our Bodies, Our Selves,* the women put to rest the common belief that the less a patient knew, the better.

Technology drove the last nail in the coffin of doctor-dominated decision making. Transplants, artificial feeding, the ventilator/respirator, and other new lifesavers raised the question to such heights that it couldn't be avoided: "When is enough enough?"

And increasingly, patients became aware, as Mrs. M did, that they bring to the doctor-patient conference something just as important as the physician's vast and amazing medical background: Their knowledge of their own amazing and vastly complex selves.

Just Say No

It's a strange turnabout.

Our right to say "no" to death-prolonging technology has been getting stronger year by year—in the hospital.

Meanwhile, that privilege has dwindled to nothing in our own homes. If we dial 911 for somebody whose heart has stopped, the paramedics are required by law to try to jump-start it. Whether it makes sense or not. Whether the patient would have wanted it or not. Of all the hundreds of city, county, and regional emergency systems, there are only twenty-three (as of last year) that don't require the medics to give cardiopulmonary resuscitation (CPR) in those situations. Only two of the fifty states—Montana and New York—give the paramedics some discretion about all-out CPR.

Most older people know this. Horror stories abound on the grapevine.

One doctor, a veteran of forty years of emergency medicine, was so worried that he had the international symbol for "No CPR" tattooed on his chest, right over his heart. An acquaintance of mine thought he was prepared, too. But it didn't help. He was over ninety years old and hadn't been well for months. The last few days, he hadn't been able to get out of bed. But, if he was going to die, he wanted to go out with dignity—at home, and without having his dying unnaturally prolonged. He had signed a Durable Power of Attorney for Health Care Decisions—the simple paper that designated someone to speak for him in case he became unconscious.

It was around 2:00 A.M. when his wife was awakened by a noise, and found that he had fallen, apparently trying to get out of bed. She wasn't strong enough to lift him. "Call 911," he said. By the time she got back from the phone, he had stopped breathing. She sat there, holding his hand, until the doorbell rang. The emergency medical technicians, all efficiency, unpacked the CPR paraphernalia, stripped off the old man's pajamas, and went to work. For forty-five minutes, they tried to pump life back into the failed ninety-year-old heart. She kept trying to show them the Durable Power of Attorney, trying to get them to stop, but to the EMTs she was just a distraction. Finally, they made her go into the other room and stay there. "Originally, I just wanted to get him back into bed," she said later. "He never would have wanted all that fuss."

When this happens in the hospital, the physician has already evaluated the likelihood of cardiac arrest and has asked the patient if he or she wants resuscitation in case of arrest. If the answer is "no," the doctor writes on the chart: "Do Not Resuscitate," or "DNR," or "No Code." For the EMTs, it's much more difficult. They don't know the patient. They're not given the decision-making powers of a physician. And, they have only minutes or even seconds to act.

Sadly, the scene in the home that morning need never have happened. In most states—including the one where my friends live—counties are working out a DNR order designed especially for these emergency situations. They give the paramedics permission to forgo CPR. The county where my friend died already is using such an order. But he and his wife didn't know—and neither did the EMTs who came to their house.

The document is issued by the Department of Emergency Medical Services of the county, and has room for the patient's and a doctor's signatures, and for the medical diagnosis. By signing it, the patient states:

"I understand that DNR means that if my heart stops, or my breathing stops, no medical treatment will be started or continued.

"I understand that DNI means that if I stop breathing I will not have a breathing tube placed into my airway.

"I understand that this DNR/DNI (do not intubate) Authorization will not prevent me from obtaining other emergency medical care by paramedics or at the direction of a physician.

"I understand that I may change my DNR/DNI Authorization at any time.

"I give permission for this information to be given to paramedics, doctors, nurses, or other health care personnel as necessary to implement any DNR/DNI Authorization."

You may not be at the stage of life where you want such a document. Most of the time 911 is called, every procedure of the paramedics is a welcome one. But if you're among the many who fear a frantic and futile scene when your time has come, now is the time to call your county Emergency Medical Services department. Ask if they have a special DNR order available.

And if not, why not.

Trial of the Century

The phrase, "trial of the century," took a bruising in the last years of the last century.

"Trial of the century" reverberated grandly in the marble walls of the U.S. Capitol, and the hand-held mikes of various folks with wind-blown hair, "reporting live" on O. J.'s murder case. But it's likely that more lives are directly affected by the Scopes "monkey trial" of 1925, for example. It still affects all of us who profit from open education and research. Or, the Nuremberg war crimes trials after World War II; they established patient consent for human research. My own nominee for trial of the century would be the Karen Ann Quinlan case, held in Morristown, New Jersey, in the 1970s. It asked the question, "Must we continue treating a patient who is in irreversible coma?"

Everybody who has been under a doctor's care, and everybody who ever expects to be, can be thankful to those who brought that case to court. Karen Quinlan's parents and their young lawyer faced money and power. The New Jersey attorney general tried the case in person. But when the verdict and the appeal were all in, the groundwork was in place for:

- recognizing patients' right to make life-and-death decisions about their own bodies;
- a shift in the doctor-patient relationship, toward a more equal role for the patient;
- ending the tradition that a physician must never give up, even when the treatment's only result was continued suffering;
- the hospital ethics committee, first of thousands—protecting patients and staff in nearly every hospital in the country.

This all began on tax day in April 1975. Karen Quinlan was twenty-one years old, depressed and out of work; her employer had "downsized" to save money a year earlier. During a birthday party for a friend at a bar, Karen collapsed. By the time the ambulance arrived, she had stopped breathing several times, and was in a coma. Doctors fought to bring her out of it. But, after weeks of testing and consultations, they told Joe and Julia Quinlan that their daughter would not wake up again.

The parents were devout Catholics with an active faith. They prayed for a miracle. Joe, a warehouse foreman active in the Knights of Columbus, was the last of the family to accept the doctors' verdict. Once he had done that, there seemed to be one logical step: let his daughter go to the life after death the family believed in, rather than remain suspended between life and death.

Karen weighed 50 pounds, was curled tightly in a fetal ball, and was fed by plastic tubes. After a bout with pneumonia, she had an artificial ventilator helping her breathe. Joe and Julia wrote Doctors Arshad Javed and Robert Morse, authorizing them to shut off the ventilator. But the doctors feared a malpractice suit or murder charges. The strong tradition of medicine was never to stop treating the patient until death took the decision out of your hands. Joe Quinlan became a crusader, not because it was his nature, but because he loved his daughter and wanted her freed. He sued to be named Karen's guardian, with the intent of withdrawing treatment. He did it with the full backing of his parish priest, Fr. Tom Trapasso, and officials of the archdiocese.

The media were there from as far away as Tokyo and London; *Newsweek* featured "The Girl in the Coma" on its cover.

The Quinlans and young Paul Armstrong, their attorney, argued that freedom of religion and the right of self-determination should give Karen freedom. Arguing that life is the ultimate good and must never be abandoned were the state, the country prosecutor, the court-appointed guardian for Karen, her doctors, and the hospital.

The Quinlans lost.

Judge Robert Muir Jr.'s decision echoed medical tradition: "A patient is placed, or places himself, in the care of a physician with the expectation that he (the physician) will do everything that is known to modern medicine, to protect his patient's life." To give up was unthinkable. Julia Quinlan told the press, "We still hope other Karens will be helped. The issue must be decided." The appeal to the State Supreme Court took months. Finally, in March 1976, the justices ruled that Joe could be his daughter's guardian—and end her treatment if he wished. It was the first Supreme Court ruling in favor of a "right to die."

The court also proposed that future cases be kept out of the courts, and be examined instead by ethics committees. Within six years, forty-eight states would affirm patients' right to refuse treatment. Hospitals now estimate that 80 percent of those who die there have refused unwanted treatment. They may not know about the trial of November 1975, but they are, in Julia Quinlan's words, "other Karens"—and in debt to the courageous Quinlan family.

Part Eleven | Issues to Ponder

A Slippery Slope?

The practice of selling human organs to people who need a transplant is nothing new. But doing it legally? That's new.

More than a quarter of a century before the old millennium ended, medicine learned how to suppress the body's natural tendency to reject organs from somebody else. Soon after, a New Jersey man put a classified ad in the *Bergen Record*, offering $25,000 for a transplantable kidney to save his life. There have been rumors of quieter deals, ever since people with kidney disease caught on to the fact that every healthy person has two kidneys—and can usually live on one.

News stories out of South America told us that gangs were kidnapping people off the street, putting them under an anesthetic, and then returning them to the street a few days later, unchanged except for the typical kidney donor's scar around the waist. And China gave us all a lesson in the workings of a free-market economy when the government began selling organs on demand to people from the industrialized nations.

Several anti-government journalists reported that patients in need of a transplant could find a contact in Hong Kong who could deliver, on a given date, an organ that was a tissue-match for the customer. The going rate: $40,000, not counting the surgeon's charge for installation. The organs purportedly came from prisoners on Death Row, who waited not only for their appeals to run out, but also for a customer whose tissues matched.

In the mid-1980s, the National Organ Transplant Act classified human organs as a national resource, and made it illegal to sell them.

Why these bizarre tales and criminal measures? The answer is simple: There are about 64,000 people in the United States (for example) who need transplants—and in 1998 there were only 5,749 donors. That was a 6 percent rise over the year before, but even with multiple organs from the same donor, you can see that there aren't anywhere near enough to go around.

That's what prompted Pennsylvania's health officials in 1999 to try offering money to families who agree to organ donation for their newly dead relatives. Pennsylvania has begun offering about $300 worth of assistance with the donor's funeral expenses. The money will be paid to the funeral home, to avoid the appearance of actually buying organs. But, the fact is, Pennsylvania is the first state to offer monetary incentives of any kind to families trying to make up their minds about donation. The experiment will be observed by a panel of bioethicists. Other states are watching the Pennsylvania experiment, ready to adopt it if there is a significant rise in the number of organ donors. The debate over Pennsylvania's audacious venture began heating up immediately. Here are some of the issues:

- Is it legal? A 1985 federal law declares that donor organs belong to the nation—a resource we hold in common, like the air. The law therefore forbids any sale of organs. On the other hand, the donor's surgical expenses are usually paid in full. Why not include the funeral costs?
- Doesn't this put the poor at a further disadvantage, since they would be more vulnerable to cash incentives? The transplant system, despite attempts to make it more just, still favors the wealthy. They have the time, can travel to surgery sites, and can afford the best health insurance.
- In order to get the funeral money, would the patient's family be less likely to disclose anything in his or her medical history that would rule out donation?
- Might the payment be the first step on a slippery slope that leads to a situation nobody wants: cash for organs?

- Is $300 a drop in the bucket? Have you looked at funeral costs lately? Three hundred dollars won't be enough for an unpainted pine box and a minister ordained by that Web site that sells degrees for $10.

The surgeon, the consultants, and the hospital, meanwhile, will cut up a six-figure pie. If Pennsylvania really wants to offer an incentive, to the donor's family, let it be enough to cover most of the expense of a simple funeral. That would be a real incentive. And, that would be a death with dignity.

The Gift

On Sunday the pastor asked not only for the offering, but our spare body parts as well.

It was Organ Donor Sunday, and he turned the pulpit over to a seventy-two-year-old Roman Catholic layman, who had a pretty compelling Thanksgiving sermon for us. He introduced himself as Gene Downs, and in six minutes of plain talk, nothing elegant, he taught us all something deep about old age, youth, and the organ donor's gift of life.

"I'm a retired Navy vet," he said, "and I've been in good health most of my life. One day I was working for the Navy along the coast, and I had a slight heart attack. At least I thought it was slight. So I told my friend and he said, 'You better go see a doctor.'

"So I went to see a doctor and he gave me a prescription for a little bottle of nitroglycerin. And he says, 'If the pain ever comes back again between your shoulder blades, you can take it.'

"While I was at the pharmacy, I had the pain, so I took the pill and broke out in a cold sweat. Ended up in the hospital. This young doc came in, and he said, 'You need a bypass.' So the next morning I had a double bypass.

"You understand, I was always very active in sports and everything. I thought I was in pretty good health."

He thought wrong. Not long after the bypass surgery, Downs had another heart attack.

"When I went in, the doctor said. 'Well, you better retire' "—Gene Downs was already in his sixties, so he took retirement from a lifetime in the Navy and moved to Sacramento.

"And one day I went into heart failure. And I was back in the hospital where I was before. And, my doctor said, 'Did you ever think about a heart transplant? You got a bad heart.'

"I said, 'Who, me?' I was already doing a lot of volunteer work with street people downtown, working with St. Vincent dePaul, and over at the Cathedral. Helping underprivileged people, you know, and he said, 'No, you better see the transplant people.' I went to see the transplant people, and I went before a review board. Took all the tests, psychology and everything. And they said, 'Sorry, you're too old.' They weren't going to give me a heart."

Over the new two years Downs had two more open heart operations and multiple angioplasty procedures—the kind where they use a tiny balloon to open clogged arteries.

"And they weren't going to give me a heart."

"So I belonged to a group called 'Sharing and Caring.' We worked out of St. Philomene's, helping sick people, all denominations, helping out, and praying for one another. So we were all there one day and I said, 'Well, I'm gonna get a heart.'

"And what happens? I have a really, really bad heart attack. They put me in a bed, and I never got out of the bed for twenty-two days. And after about two weeks, Dr. Paul Kelly came in and he said, 'Gene, we've reviewed your case, and we're gonna give you a beeper—for a heart transplant.'

"But he said, "You've very sick; if you don't get a heart within a week you're gonna be dead; we're gonna take you out of here on a gurney.'

"Five days later, a nurse's aide came in and she says, "Your coordinator's on the phone.' Well, I knew I was going to get a heart.

"So that night I got the heart of a fifteen-year-old boy. I was the oldest man—I was sixty-six at the time. I'll be seventy-three when my heart anniversary comes up next month, and it'll be more than seven years. And, on Christmas Eve, I'm gonna get to meet the boy's family. The mother would like to give a present to his siblings, to meet the man who's got her son's heart." Downs stopped, obviously moved.

"Excuse me; it's very hard. I felt very guilty—a sixty-six-year-old man gettin' a fifteen-year-old boy's heart. That's my story. And remember this: There are 66,000 people out there waiting for organs.

"But now, because of me and a couple of other old guys, they're giving organs to those up into their seventies. Thank you."

*   *   *

The week he gave this talk, the papers say, members of Congress were breaking an agreement with the Administration for a fairer way of distributing organs. And in Baltimore, the United Network for Organ Sharing was wrangling over the proposed change, stalling reform for another three months or so. A. Watson Bell, the public member, rebuked the board for its paralysis, in language Gene Downs would have appreciated: "Shame on me and shame on us and shame on our government and shame on the transplant community.

"People are dying who shouldn't have to die."

Arithmetic Lesson

Puns are fun, but that "sin tax" label for the taxes on cigarettes—to help pay for health care reform—has to go. It just doesn't work. It leaves the door open to the conclusion that the tax would be a punitive move, based on our Puritan disapproval of something enjoyed by so many people. To turn around an old Mae West line, "Badness has nothing to do with it."

The judgmental approach isn't appropriate, even if it were helpful. Most of us do things that hurt our bodies, from pigging out on French fries to running nonstop on adrenalin. Nor does it work. Somebody else's disapproval isn't a curative force for people struggling to break an addiction. Most important, the "cigareets and whisky and wild, wild women" approach trivializes the issue. It masks the harsh reality of cigarette smoking—its impact on lives, its cost to the U.S. medical system.

Some reminders:

Illicit drugs like heroin and cocaine, for all the publicity they get, kill between 5,000 and 10,000 people a year in the United States. Cigarettes, by the most conservative estimates, kill 350,000.

Cigarettes kill more people than AIDS. More than alcohol.
More than automobile accidents. More than fires.
More than homicide and suicide.
More than all those causes put together, plus illegal drugs.
Fifty percent more than all those put together.

"Even well-educated professionals are often incredulous when confronted with this simple arithmetic fact," according to Professor Kenneth Warner, the senior scientific editor of the 1989 *Surgeon General's Report on Smoking and Health*. But, he says, "Smoking is by far the nation's leading cause of preventable, premature death."

Cost to the U.S. health care system: At least $50 billion a year.

The toll includes 20 percent of the deaths from heart disease, 30 percent of all cancer deaths, and 80 percent of the deaths from chronic obstructive lung disease. Cancer researcher and biochemistry chairman Bruce Ames of the University of California, Berkeley, has suggested that if it weren't for tobacco smoking, the overall death rates for cancer in this country would be falling, not rising.

If cigarettes were pickup trucks, they would long since have been recalled from the streets because of their danger.

A conference organized by the American Medical Association to curb the use of tobacco recommended the following:

- More federal prosecutors should consider fraud charges against the tobacco companies, for fooling consumers about the health effects.
- Federal agencies should sponsor a stop-smoking campaign aimed especially at women—among whom smoking is on the rise. No coincidence: Lung cancer has passed breast cancer as a cause of death among U.S. women. More than 53,000 women die of lung cancer each year.
- Government at all levels should ban smoking in schools, public facilities, and workplaces.
- Raise the federal excise tax on cigarettes to $2 a pack, and encourage the states to raise their taxes on tobacco too.

Despite the strength of the addiction and the power of advertising, tobacco companies are selling fewer cigarettes in the United States than they did. But that raises a problem that could be more trouble for the

President than getting a bigger per-pack tax passed: American tobacco companies are making up for dwindling sales here by vigorously pushing nicotine overseas. And they've been doing it with the support of the U.S. government. Rep. Henry Waxman (D-Calif.) has compared it to England's exports of opium to China in the 1830s, to improve its balance of trade with that silk-and tea-producing nation. The government was involved, under presidents Reagan and Bush, because of the power of the thirty or so tobacco-state members of Congress. Carla Hills, Bush's trade representative, energetically fought the trade barriers against U.S. cigarettes, and energetically denied that there was a moral problem. "As long as cigarettes remain a legal commodity in the United States and abroad, there is no legal basis to deny cigarette manufacturers assistance in gaining market access," her office told the General Accounting Office.

So, for six years in the 1980s, the number of cigarettes we sent abroad doubled, to 100 billion a year. With horrendous potential results. In 1989, the World Health Organization gathered a panel of consultants to calculate how many people now living will be killed by tobacco if present rates of smoking continue. Richard Peto, an Oxford University epidemiologist, reported the result to the Seventh World Congress on Tobacco and Health, held in Perth, Australia. The figure: 500 million people now living are doomed to die of tobacco-caused diseases. More than 200 million of these are children or teenagers today.

Meanwhile, back in the U.S., Congressman Henry A. Waxman looks at the figures and says, "Until we improve control of tobacco use it is going to be difficult to control medical costs."

Estimated cost to the nation's health care system is now $50 billion a year. That—not the tongue-in-cheek idea of taxing sin—is the hard argument for raising the federal excise tax on cigarettes and continuing the lawsuits against manufacturers.

Defining Disasters

Do you prefer your disasters in brief, intense doses, or spread out over time? Concentrated manageably in one place, or scattered across thousands of miles? Natural calamities raise questions about our response to human need. If nothing else, they remind us how irrational our reaction can be.

Consider some examples:

In one month, fifty to sixty people died from a California quake; thousands suddenly became homeless, and hundreds ended up in the hospital. Meanwhile, in the Midwest and East, more than twice as many people were dying in a big freeze and snowstorm. Thousands were hurt in crashes on icy roads. The earthquake brought shock, sympathy, and the top headlines in most media outlets. The reaction to the storm—spread across many states, over days instead of minutes—was softer; smaller headlines, even (in the sun states, at least) a tinge of amusement.

Reaction to the quake included TV reporters' endlessly asking people in L.A.: "Do you think all these disasters will make you want to move out of California?" If any of them asked the same question of the folks stuck in the snow back East, we missed it. A freezing blizzard that kills 130 people is not a disaster as serious, apparently, as a quake that kills fifty.

Other disasters are equally tragic—but draw hardly any headlines at all. The main difference seems to be the time span.

- The number of children killed by guns since 1979 passed the number of soldiers killed in the Vietnam War, according to a report by the Children's Defense Fund.
- Hundreds of thousands of people stood in soup lines and slept in the street or in public shelters—victims not of Mother Nature but of long-term calamities like mental illness or unemployment.
- Just as thoroughly wounded as if they'd been caught in a blizzard or an earthquake, millions of chronically ill men, women and children struggled to get through each day. For them, no helicopter rescue, no FEMA, no headlines.
- More subtle than a broken leg but harder to heal, the trauma of sexism, racism, homophobia, and other bigotry kept taking its toll. For example, these figures just released: One-third of all African Americans live below the poverty line; 12 percent of African Americans can't get jobs.

- The AIDS epidemic wipes out women and men in the prime of youth, with the toll well over 200,000. But, the idea of a coordinated federal approach, of seeing this as an emergency requiring intense response, seems as far away as it was under Ronald Reagan.

We accept this difference in attitudes as "human nature." It doesn't surprise us that we get more excited about short-term, localized disasters than about long-term, nationwide tragedies. It's always been that way.

But, why?

Is it the complexity? Would we get more excited if an emergency task force could swoop into an area and mop up after tragedies like poverty, violence, and hatred? Many doctors find it hard to stay interested in patients with chronic illness, because it leaves even the best physicians helpless and frustrated. Is the same thing behind our society's response to chronic calamity? Or is it because the causes of long-term ills tend to be so vague and complex? When we're frostbitten at 30 below and lose some toes, the cause is something we can understand. The causes of poverty, on the other hand, are not only incredibly complex, but are oversimplified and distorted. They lend themselves to deluded thinking—the kind that lets the rest of us off the hook. While the earthquake homeless are seen as helpless victims (for example), the long-term homeless "really prefer to be homeless." They "like the outdoor life," or are "free spirits refusing to be tied down."

The poor, we convince ourselves, are that way because they have done something wrong and are being punished by God. It's a judgmental self-delusion that lurks deep in our national subconscious, whether we admit it or not. Much of the rhetoric about welfare is based not on fact but on this kind of thinking. So, we're left with one of the great conundrums: Acute disasters unify us as a people; we rally 'round, we empathize.

But chronic disasters divide us into hostile camps: roughly, those who believe the victims had it coming to them, versus those who believe we could rally 'round, helping one another in long-term disasters just as in those that are over in seconds.

Freedom Isn't Free

The grizzled bikers looked like extras from a Brando movie, but their main interest was a philosophical question: To what extent should government limit our freedom, in order to protect us from ourselves? Gunning their engines and swaggering for the cameras, several hundred motorcycle riders had gathered at the California state capitol to denounce a new mandatory helmet law.

"I should have the choice if I want to get my brains splattered all over the street," one bearded and booted biker told a TV reporter. A middle-aged man in full Hells Angels regalia told a reporter, "It's just another nick, another chipping away at my rights. Pretty soon they're going to be telling us what to wear."

But like most of us, he had a mixed agenda; it wasn't all human rights: "Besides," he said, "I have a certain image to uphold, and I don't want people thinking I look funny."

Our answer to the protect-you-from-yourself question is mixed, too. We have to buckle up. We're supposed to abide by the speed limit. We need a doctor's prescription to get certain drugs; others we aren't supposed to have at all. They tell us this makes us safer, and it does. But the stronger argument, I suspect, is that it keeps us from hurting other people. I wonder whether we'd have a law against driving under the influence, for example, if drunk drivers killed only themselves. Seat belts, like helmets on bikers, protect the wearer—but also save on medical bills that somebody else might have ended up paying.

In 1990, some 18,000 California motorcyclists managed to get themselves hurt on the road, and 562 were killed. The Highway Patrol thinks helmets would have saved 150 to 200 of those lives.

Unless they're willing to pay their own medical bills, it makes sense to require the helmets, and to have seat-belt and speed laws.

But, wait. If the rule is, "Pay for your own foolishness, or give it up," we're not consistent about enforcing it. A second piece of pie or a large order of fries can be as potentially fatal, alas, as riding without a helmet. Cancer and heart disease, no less than AIDs, can result from conscious acts. And who pays the medical bills? All of us, through taxes and insurance premiums. But nobody is talking about giving a ticket to everyone caught on the street wearing more than 250 pounds of fat. Or of mandatory testing for high cholesterol.

On the other hand, some people are as serious about tobacco as about helmets. In Lansing, a few days after the bikers' failed PR effort in Sacramento, the governor of Michigan got a phone call from former surgeon general Everett Koop.

Koop was speaking for a coalition of fifty-seven groups, including the American Heart Association and the American Cancer Society, who want Michigan to double the tax on tobacco products. In a follow-up letter, Koop said, "Tobacco use is the single most important preventable cause of death in our society." He said the tax would be "one of the most effective strategies to improve the health of our citizens."

Can't argue with that. But you can bet the smokers, like the bikers, will feel that they're being discriminated against. And, they may be right. We require helmets but not healthy diets. We tax cigarettes, but don't ban them. We ban pot, but not booze. What's the operating principle? Maybe it's just plain pragmatic: We regulate what we think we can enforce. Some bikers get saved, despite themselves. And some heavy eaters (and smokers and drinkers) leave us early because of themselves.

And leave us with the check, too.

Part Twelve | Violence as a Health Issue

Ignoring Violence

This is about a sickness that can't be cured in a hospital. It's a form of selective blindness, that clearly sees certain kinds of violence but is oblivious to others just as dangerous. I began to recognize it in the heat and tumult of Mississippi, working as a civil rights worker in the mid-1960s. I met a man whose gnarled hands were frozen into loose fists. We were eating hamburgers together—it was his first—and his hands couldn't unclench enough to grip the bun.

I remember thinking they were like the hands of a pool hustler in one of those movies where the hero gets caught and is forced to grip his cue while his knuckles are broken by blows. But the violence that maimed my new friend took longer than that: nearly seventy years of gripping a hoe, in a world whose only interest in him—and the only choice ever open to him—was as a cotton chopper.

- When the economy calls for it, hundreds of thousands of men and women are laid off in the midst of a culture that says people are of worth only when they are producing. The incidence of wife-battering and child abuse always rises with the jobless rate, and we rightly deplore those acts. But, the employer who brought on the layoffs, whether it was by moving his plant to another country to save on the payroll, or just cutting back to boost the dividends, is also committing a violent act, disrupting lives and shattering homes. We choose not to see that violence.

- We'll disparage what we call union violence—even lawful strikes—and ignore the silent violence of union-busting, of power that keeps men and women working without a contract, and slows negotiations to a caterpillar's pace.
- A five-year-old lies in a bed at home, blind and so crippled from cerebral palsy that he can't turn himself over. Heavy blows from a blunt weapon could have produced the same result, but the act of violence that put him there was the stroke of a pen in Washington, slashing federal funds for prenatal clinics.
- The late comedian Godfrey Cambridge used to tell about his frustration, night after night when his show was over, of trying to get a taxi to take him uptown in Manhattan. The driver would slow, and then when he saw Cambridge was black, would speed on past. One night Cambridge tore the door off a cab that was trying to pull away. His violent act made all the papers and the TV news. But not the silent, brutal violence of the blows to Cambridge's mind, repeated night after night, from strangers who saw his skin and said, "Not in my cab."
- President Bush came on TV and tut-tutted the first Rodney King beating verdict, and then roundly denounced the rioting that followed in Los Angeles. But we're all blind to the deeper violence when the White House and Congress play politics with the stuff of people's lives. Refusing to deal with the health care crisis is maiming more bodies, killing more people, than all the power-crazed cops or greedy looters in the country. It's institutional violence. It's violence that takes years, instead of thirty-second action clips.
- A while back, a series of bombings hit dozens of clinics that performed safe and legal abortions. The president of that day did not go on TV to denounce this, and his Bureau of Alcohol, Tobacco, and Firearms determined, with the help of the FBI, that there was no pattern, no conspiracy here. Must be coincidence, they said.
- The shrill harridans who invade the privacy of women in trouble who have come to abortion clinics have not been denounced. On the contrary. This assault of venom and vituperation, and sometimes of physical abuse, is encouraged by government pandering to the religious right on the issue of women's choice.

- Joe Morgan, courtly baseball commentator, a Hall of Fame player, and one of the finest men in the game, found himself jerked from his car, and spread-eagled for search, for no other reason than that he was black and in a "good" neighborhood. We heard about it because he's a public figure; most urban African Americans have had similar experiences. Public violence, such as riots, are not justified by the less visible, ongoing violence. But, you can't understand the one without seeing the other.
- Fearful and sick-souled young guys drive in from the suburbs to beat up gay men and lesbians. Most of us ignore the fact that these perverted acts of violence are increasing each year. We've even more determined to ignore the connection between these insecure, swaggering punks and the panderers who give them permission to act—including the churches.

But you and I can't judge them too harshly. They'd never get away with it, if you and I weren't so studiously ignoring the violence too.

Home Sweet Home?

It was murder for a couple of weeks, here in our medium-sized Western city. Four men killed their wives, ex-wives, or woman friends. One murdered his ex-wife, their two little girls, and the ex-wife's boyfriend. It wasn't brought on by the heat. These killings—I almost said "shootings," but we all know that guns don't kill people—took place during mild weather for us, the low nineties. As a matter of fact, these grisly deaths were nothing unusual. Whatever sickness drives a person to beat up or kill a spouse or a kid, it's a worldwide epidemic.

Then Secretary of State Madeline Albright said, "Today around the world, appalling abuses are being committed against women, from domestic violence, to dowry murders, to mutilation, to forcing young girls into prostitution.

"Some say all this is cultural and there's nothing we can do about it. I say it's criminal, and we have a responsibility to stop it."

These journeys of courage start with a single step, of course, and that includes recognizing that the United States is at least as much of a problem as it is a solution. Dr. James O. Mason, then head of the Public Health Service, asked a 1992 conference on family violence: "Why are we more violent than other peoples, with a white male homicide rate, in a recent international study, well over twice that of Scotland, our nearest competitor?"

Bonnie Campbell, chief of the attorney general's division administering the Women Against Violence Act, points out that while 55,000 American men were dying in Vietnam, "more than that number of American women were killed by batterers during that same period of time."

These truths are self-evident, but they're easy to ignore:

- We're still a world of patriarchal societies, where women's word and worth are valued less than men's.
- We're still a violent society, and we condone or even encourage some forms of mayhem.

Put the two together and you have the serious health problem called spouse abuse. You have a society in which men can batter women with impunity, whether they're famous football heroes or not.

Patriarchy? If you doubt it, consider this homely example: Wife-beating goes up drastically in areas where there have been heavy employee layoffs. The anger and frustration are predictable—but why the target? Why don't these disturbed men beat up their bosses? Or the guys who didn't get laid off?

Answer: Because bosses and buddies are not acceptable targets, and a woman is. No matter how long a way we've come, baby, woman is a chattel in the eyes of many men ("Who gives this woman . . . ?").

Violence? Dr. Mason *might have* asked questions like these:

What is the impact of TV violence, including wrestling and football? Of telling a boy to "be a man" and settle a dispute with his fists? Of being the only industrial nation that tries to stop murder by killing the perpetrator? Of making "tomboy" a compliment and "sissy" a put-down?

The result is a health issue, Mason said: "One-fifth to one-third of all women are physically abused during their lifetime. Ten percent of the time the injury is serious enough to require hospitalization or emergency room treatment."

There was more.

Homeless: "25-50 percent of homeless families are headed by women who left home to escape domestic violence."

Murder: "Half of the murdered women in the United States are killed by a current or former partner."

An answer to the half-baked question, "Why don't they just leave?": "Women who are divorced, separated, or otherwise estranged from their partners are at the highest risk of assault."

Meanwhile, most of the country preferred to look the other way.

Shelter operators have to turn away two women for every one they have room for. Government aid for agencies helping victims has dropped by 35 percent in fifteen years. Three women a day are murdered by their partners.

A sign: In June, 1992, the National Domestic Violence Hotline, which had been receiving as many as 10,000 calls a month, had to shut down for lack of money.

It was four years before the new Women Against Violence Act restored such programs.

To Bonnie Campbell, it was a serious step. "If you think about it, being a prisoner in a home where someone controls every move you make isn't substantially different than being a POW, or being in a concentration camp in Nazi Germany, or being killed by Stalin's henchmen. Violence is fundamental. Living your life free of it is a fundamental right."

A Dubious Analogy

The Klan had lined up across the front of the little white frame church, standing just far enough apart that we could walk between them and go on in. If we felt like it.

These weren't the Klansmen you know from the documentaries, with pointy-headed bed sheets and hysterical rhetoric. The Klan in Natchez on that night in 1965 wore hard hats, and each had a billy club. None of them said a word; the silence was deafening. They just stood there in a line across the sidewalk leading into the church, watching each of us as we arrived.

Despite the intimidation, it was standing-room-only inside. Fed-up black residents were seeking a few of the amenities the white section of Natchez took for granted: paved streets, for example, and sewers. Police protection, instead of intimidation.

Five nights before, after a rally in the church, twenty-five people had left to march peacefully to City Hall and leave a list of requests.

They never got there.

A block from the church, city police had arrested them, packed them into an old bus, and sent them 190 miles north to Parchman Penitentiary.

The next night, it had taken two buses to take the marchers to Parchman. Every night, more marchers. Meanwhile, a bomb under the seat of his pickup had killed one of the church members.

On the night in question, the first few people were back from the penitentiary—a handful of the elderly and the sick, released early.

It was a classic freedom rally, a combination of political rally and revival service. African Americans of all ages, with a handful of us northern whites. The mood was hopeful, fearful, angry, determined. We sang a spiritual one moment and a freedom song the next.

One of the speakers that night was a woman in her eighties who had just come back from Parchman that day. She told of the assaults on dignity: being strip-searched and herded, naked, into crowded cells, with the male guards always looking on. Of a pail for a toilet, and of being issued one square of toilet paper per day.

Others told of similar indignities, and when they were finished, a pastor asked: "All right now, who'll march tonight?" As if on signal, everybody turned and looked out the open rear door. A police bus was there, backed up to the door. There was a moment's silence, and then a woman's voice began a slow tune, followed by the others:

> *"O freedom! O freedom!*
> *O freedom over me!*
> *And, before I'll be a slave,*

I'll be buried in my grave,
And go home to my Lord and be free!"

Before the first verse was over, the woman who had started the song was on her way, singing, toward the door. Half the church followed her out the door. I didn't know her name, but I recognized her: She was the elderly woman who had come back from the penitentiary that morning.

*   *   *

What brought back this memory, many years later, was a newspaper story about the tactics being used these days to stop legal abortions.

"All we're doing," the leader of one anti-abortion group had told the press: "is what the civil rights movement did in the 1960s."

It made my hair stand on end.

The civil rights movement was built on *nonviolent* action, not on harassment and mayhem. We put ourselves in positions where, if there was to be violence, we would be the victims, not the perpetrators.

We were the spat-upon, not the spitters.

We took our stand—and, if necessary, our blows—in hopes that the world would see the difference, and recognize violence and bigotry for what they are.

The black people of Natchez had a right to be morally indignant. Tourists came from around the world to see the great pre-War mansions of Natchez, but the sewers in the black neighborhoods were open ditches along dirt streets. Schools were a joke and police protection nil. The median wage was $3 a day, and the better-paying jobs were closed to African Americans.

But, they didn't call up the mayor's family and threaten him. They didn't burn down City Hall. They didn't bomb anybody, not even with stink bombs. They didn't push, shove, or scream at the nearest white person.

Even when their leader was killed by that bomb in his pickup truck, there was no retaliation.

The truth behind this was simple—a matter of ethics and integrity:

Even when you are opposing a force that you believe is morally wrong, you don't use morally questionable tactics.

The Birth of the Electric Chair

A court battle in California brought to mind one of the more bizarre moments in American science—the birth of the electric chair.

Both events, 100 years apart, have to do with that granddaddy of all oxymorons: humane execution.

In 1993, various experts testified that death in California's gas chamber is (a) swift, painless and merciful, or (b) slow, painful and cruel.

The 1880s event saw one of our great American heroes testifying on behalf of electrocution in a way that advanced his own inventions and tainted a rival's work. He was Thomas Alva Edison, already father of the phonograph and the electric light, and the man who eventually would give us the movies. During the early 1880s, Edison had been putting all his energy into a system for delivering electricity. His lightbulb had captured the country's imagination, but it was useless without juice. Edison controlled—and profited from—every segment of the system, from generators and cables to motors and lightbulbs. Downtown New York City was his first big customer; there was another fortune to be made if other cities signed on. Unfortunately, direct current couldn't be sent more than a few blocks; most users had to have their own noisy generator. Still, DC seemed to be the best thing around, and the magic name of Edison made the public ignore the weaknesses.

The threat to this dream of profit came from another successful inventor with big money to spend: George Westinghouse, developer of the railroad air brake. By the mid-1880s, his Westinghouse Electric Co. was pushing a system of delivering electricity based on alternating current, or AC. AC could be transmitted for many miles; generators could be bigger and fewer, and built far out of earshot—even out of town. Soon, Westinghouse was competing with Edison for the franchise in dozens of cities. The contest between the two stubborn and proud tycoon-inventors has been called "the War of the Currents."

Fear became a weapon. Edison believed AC was far more dangerous than DC, and soon started a campaign to make AC illegal. He flooded cities with pamphlets warning of AC's danger to families. An aide, H. P. Brown, began experimenting with alternating current "electricide," killing dogs and cats brought to him by local kids who got a quarter per pet. Brown said he was doing research on the dangers of AC, but made sure the press got to watch a killing or two.

Up in Albany, the governor saw the accounts. The state had been looking for a better form of execution than hanging, which had been known to cause slow strangulation if the rope was too loose, and to tear the prisoner's head off his body if it was too tight. The Commission on Humane Executions asked Edison for data, but he turned them down; he didn't believe in capital punishment. Later, after thinking it over, he gave his full backing to execution by wire, strongly affirming it as the most humane form of execution. He was even kind enough to recommend the best generator for the job: "Alternating machines, manufactured principally in this country by George Westinghouse."

The Legislature soon passed a bill making "electricide" the official state form of execution.

The person who viewed all this with the most interest was William Kemmler, twenty-eight, a convicted killer who was next up for execution. Kemmler's lawyer tried to stop the execution, arguing that using electricity would be cruel and unusual punishment. Edison testified for the state, assuring the judge that electrocution would be painless. That was all the judge needed to hear.

Kemmler was strapped into the chair on August 6, 1890. The first jolt of alternating current lasted 17 seconds. Kemmler continued struggling. A second jolt lasted more than a minute—until smoke was seen rising from the body. It was, the *New York Times* said, "an awful spectacle, far worse than hanging."

The state commissioner on human executions saw it differently. It was, he said, "the grandest success of the age."

Ira Flatow, the science reporter whose lively 1992 book, *They All Laughed* has the best account of the Current War, writes: "Kemmler was more than a victim of his crime; he was a pawn (in) a vicious battle between two giants of the industry . . . to control the future of electric generation."

Edison's strange behavior is a good reminder that homicide, whether in war, in the gas chamber, or on the mean streets is likely to be the result of politics, emotion, and greed—not the reasoned intent with which we like to credit ourselves.

The Seamless Garment

The late Cardinal Bernardin made a return visit the other day.

He came in the person of Pope John Paul II, asking Catholics to add capital punishment to the list of sins that cheapen human life.

It was the Cardinal, an untimely loss to cancer in 1998, who had frequently nudged people of his faith—along with the rest of us and, perhaps, his pope—to adopt "a seamless garment" in their beliefs about life-and-death issues.

American bishops and their priests spoke early and often against abortion, euthanasia, and assisted suicide, but went mute on the subject of the death penalty.

Speaking in St. Louis, the pope said: "I renew the appeal . . . for a consensus to end the death penalty which is both cruel and unnecessary."

He welcomed "the increasing recognition that the dignity of human life must never be taken away, even in the case of someone who has done great evil. Modern society has the means of protecting itself, without definitively denying criminals the chance to reform."

He pointed out that 500 criminals had been executed in the United States since the death penalty was reinstated in 1977.

Americans support the death penalty by somewhere between 65 and 80 percent, depending on how the question is asked. But if the question is preceded by a condition—"If you could be sure the sentence would be life without possibility of parole"—the support for the death penalty drops to below 50 percent.

Cardinal Bernardin wasn't the only one to notice and criticize the inconsistency in being pro-life on one issue and pro-death on another.

British physician Richard H. Nicholson wrote in the bioethics journal, the *Hastings Center Report*, that when Parliament last debated capital punishment (in the late-1980s), "those members who voted unsuccessfully for a return of capital punishment were virtually identical to the group that had a few months earlier voted to ban abortions.

"It might be a very fruitful field of enquiry to examine why there is so often a close concurrence between pro-life views and support for capital punishment."

Some see an equal inconsistency among the pro-choice advocates, many of whom oppose the death penalty but accept that some people will "kill unborn babies" by abortion. However, that definition is what divides pro-choice and anti-abortion factions. At the heart of the pro-choice stand is the belief that the fetus, while a potential human being, is not yet a human—and thus there is no murder.

Meanwhile, doctors have been arguing their own death-penalty question: Should a physician participate? The question comes up more frequently these days because, ironically, the most humane form of execution—lethal injection—is most likely to require a physician's help. Lawrence Egbert, M.D., an anesthesiologist and president of the Maryland chapter of Physicians for Social Responsibility, wrote in a 1998 issue of the Jesuit weekly, *America*: "Physicians have prescribed tranquilizers as part of the preparation for executions. We have selected intravenous sites for the injection. We, or people under our supervision, have started the intravenous injections. We have prescribed the drugs, consulted about the drugs and their doses and order of administration. We have monitored to determine death. In summary, physicians have participated in every step of executions, including the psychiatric evaluations that may lead toward an execution."

The *American Medical News* says that of the thirty-six states with death penalties, almost two-thirds have procedures that require a doctor's involvement. This happens despite the fact that the American Medical Association is adamantly opposed to physician involvement in executions.

In 1992 the AMA's Council on Ethical and Judicial Affairs ruled: "A physician, as a member of a profession dedicated to preserving life when there is hope of doing so, should not be a participant in a legally authorized execution."

Some physicians criticize the AMA for failing to condemn capital punishment altogether, rather than just its doctors' role in it. In fact, it precedes the sentences above with this one: "An individual's opinion on capital punishment is the personal moral decision of the individual."

It makes you wonder: If physicians think executions are so horrendous that they shouldn't take part in them, then why aren't they opposed to other people doing them?

Lawrence D. Egbert, M. D. says flatly: "Executing people is wrong. Having physicians participate adds to the wrong. Why does the state kill people to show others that killing people is bad?"

Study Guide

Written by John D. Schroeder

Second Opinion offers reflections on contemporary issues in bioethics. As a discussion leader, you have the opportunity to help others answer questions on a variety of issues through group dynamics. The conversations in your group may cover a variety of topics as together you ask questions and seek answers. Here are some thoughts on how to best facilitate this process.

Suggestions for Leaders

1. Read the entire book before your first group meeting. This will provide you with an overview of the material and will better equip you as a leader.
2. Distribute the book to participants before the first meeting and request they come having read the first chapter.
3. Begin each session by reviewing the main points using the chapter summary in this leader's guide.
4. Select the discussion questions and activities in advance. Feel free to change the order of the listed questions and create your own questions. Allow a set amount of time for the questions and activities.
5. Remind your participants that all questions are valid as part of the learning process. Invite them to share their thoughts, personal stories, and ideas as their comfort level dictates.

6. Some questions may be more difficult to answer than others. If you ask a question and no one responds, begin the discussion by venturing an answer yourself. Then ask for comments and other answers. Remember that some questions may have multiple answers.

7. Ask the question "Why?" or "Why do you believe that?" to help continue a discussion and give it greater depth.

8. Give everyone a chance to talk. Keep the conversation moving. You may want to direct a question at a specific person who has been quiet. "Do you have anything to add?" is a good follow-up question to another person. If the topic of conversation gets off track, move ahead by asking the next question in your leader's guide.

9. Before moving from questions to activities, ask members if they have any questions that have not been answered. Remember that as a leader, you do not have to know all the answers. Some answers will come from group members. Your role is that of facilitator, to keep the discussion moving and to encourage participation.

10. Conclude with your selected activity or a group discussion. Set aside a specific amount of time for this.

11. Be grateful and supportive. Thank members for their ideas and participation.

PART 1: DECISIONS

Chapter Summary
- There are many ways in which to help a friend or family member who is very sick.
- Advance planning can make your hospital stay smoother and safer.
- Durable Power of Attorney for Health Care gives you a voice when you are ill.
- Death is a part of life and needs to be discussed.
- The best decisions are informed decisions.

Discussion Questions

1. What new insights did you receive from reading this section?
2. Recall a time you visited a sick friend. How did it feel? Were you able to help? In what way?
3. What was a past visit to a hospital like when you were the patient? What went well and not so well?
4. What is a good basis for making medical decisions for yourself, others?
5. Have you ever talked to someone about death as a fact of life? If so, how did you feel after the conversation?
6. What does "family values" mean to you?
7. What are the benefits of talking about death?
8. What are the benefits of Durable Power of Attorney for Health Care?
9. What are the risks and costs of Durable Power of Attorney for Health Care?
10. How do bad medical decisions get made by people and doctors? List some causes.
11. What questions or concerns were raised as you read this section?
12. When is it easier to talk about death? What makes it difficult to talk about death?

Activities / Group Discussion

1. Discuss the ethics of telling the truth in medical situations and include circumstances. Look at the issue both pro and con.
2. Make a list of family values your entire group can agree on.
3. List what you feel should be some basic rights of patients.
4. List what you feel should be some basic rights of a dying person.
5. Discuss some strategies for receiving the best in health care.

PART 2: ALTERNATIVE REPRODUCTIVE TECHNOLOGY

Chapter Summary

- Technology is out-racing our wisdom on this issue.
- Technology complicates reaching a conclusion that death has occurred.

- One of the toughest ethical calls is how much effort should be made to save a premature baby.
- Moral tests complicate answering "who is a mother?"
- Gene testing presents many pros and cons for all parties involved.

Discussion Questions

1. What new insights did you receive from reading this section?
2. In your own words, explain what alternative reproductive technology means to you.
3. Why may a location be a critical principle of medical ethics?
4. What questions did the Marie Henderson case raise for you?
5. What is the newest legal sign of death?
6. What was the source of confusion in the Marie Henderson case?
7. How did the Johns Hopkins study simplify the question a little on which preemies to try and save?
8. What are some of the basic issues involved when it comes to premature births?
9. What issues complicate the question of who ought to be a mother?
10. What are some social barriers to older women having children?
11. What are some reasons multiple births are increasing?
12. What are the benefits of the two-embryo standard?

Activities / Group Discussion

1. List what's wrong and right with getting infertile people together with the best possible virtual mate.
2. Discuss some of the issues involved in gene testing.
3. List some of the centuries-old expectations of womanly behavior.
4. Create a list of the pros and cons of gene testing.
5. Discuss some of the issues raised in "May Day" regarding fertility, drugs, and clinics.

PART 3: HEALTH CARE

Chapter Summary
- Health care changes when the status quo is challenged.
- Most patients don't get the treatment they need for pain.
- Health care professionals often suffer and grieve when losing a patient.
- Heath care is now moving toward treating the whole person.
- Health care professionals are getting better at shifting gears to help a dying patient.

Discussion Questions
1. What new insights did you receive from reading this section?
2. How did Iqbal Masih make a difference?
3. What are some of the issues regarding the treatment of pain?
4. Why are some physicians reluctant to give medicine to ease pain?
5. Recall a struggle with pain in your past. Did you receive enough of the right medication? Why or why not?
6. Why do health professionals sometimes handle the issue of death so poorly?
7. Name some reasons people often prefer home care over nursing homes.
8. What did you learn from "the Spocks on Patients"?
9. Name some reasons doctors overmedicate and undermedicate.
10. In your own words, explain the idea of double effect? What is the third effect?
11. How is treatment of pain changing?
12. How do value judgments and religious beliefs influence pain treatment?

Activities / Group Discussion
1. List some signs of a good nursing home.
2. Discuss some ways to effectively communicate pain.
3. Talk to your physician about his or her philosophy in treating pain.
4. Discuss ways that doctors and patients can grieve more effectively.
5. Make a list of what you expect from your doctor when you are dying.

PART 4: DNA

Chapter Summary

- Most Americans believe that DNA research is reliable.
- Crick and Watson discovered the double helix, the shape of DNA, in 1953.
- DNA is utilized in many practical ways to solve problems in society.
- Twenty-five percent of Fortune 500 companies have used DNA testing to weed out potential employees.
- DNA has often been used to connect a person to a crime scene, or to prove there is no connection.

Discussion Questions

1. What new insights did you receive from reading this section?
2. Do you think that DNA is reliable? Why or why not?
3. Do you believe embryos are human beings? Why or why not?
4. What do you think about cloning human cells?
5. In your own words, explain the concept of DNA.
6. When did you first hear about DNA and in what context?
7. What are some of the uses of cloning that are not accepted?
8. What are some uses where cloning could be helpful?
9. Do you think the human brain can keep pace with technology? Why or why not?
10. Give your opinion on the Roy Criner case.
11. What do you think is the strongest argument against cloning human cells?
12. What factors keep people in prison who have been cleared by DNA?

Activities / Group Discussion

1. Read more about DNA at your local library.
2. Discuss the pros and cons of the FBI having a national database.
3. How can DNA be used for good? How could it be used for bad purposes?
4. Discuss how opinions get formed about DNA or cloning.
5. Would you want to be cloned? Why or why not?

PART 5: NOTEWORTHY CASES

Chapter Summary

- Genetic engineering is being used to answer many fascinating questions.
- DNA can tie a person to a crime scene or prove a person is innocent.
- As technology improves, more ethical questions arise.
- The decision of James Michener reminds us we have a choice.
- "Brain death" became part of our culture and language following the death of Robert Kennedy.

Discussion Questions

1. What new insights did you receive from reading this section?
2. What do you believe makes a case noteworthy?
3. What do you think about using DNA testing in regard to the French heir?
4. Give your reaction to the story about Charles Dickens.
5. List some of the issues raised in the Charles Dickens story.
6. Would you rather die at home or in a hospital? Why?
7. How and why have hospitals been used to hide the dying?
8. After World War II, what two things helped determine where death took place?
9. How was death further defined after the assassination of Robert Kennedy?
10. What motivates us to change our views on death and dying?
11. How have your views on death and dying changed over the years?
12. Did any of your views change as a result of this reading or discussion? Explain.

Activities / Group Discussion

1. Discuss the limits of genetic testing.
2. Discuss the possibilities of genetic testing.
3. List what you think are reasonable rules for waiting lists for organ transplants.
4. List the pros and cons of dying at home and dying at a hospital.

5. List the pros and cons of using DNA testing to screen prospective employees.

PART 6: FUTILE TREATMENT

Chapter Summary
- There is often no community standard on what health care is futile.
- Doctors are sometimes reluctant to go against family wishes.
- Futile treatment must be defined in order for health care to be reformed.
- Moral questions complicate the issue of futile treatment.
- It has been estimated that there are between 10,000 and 25,000 PVS patients on life support at any given time.

Discussion Questions
1. What new insights did you receive from reading this section?
2. In your own words, explain what "futile treatment" means to you.
3. Have you ever pushed a doctor for medicine against his or her wishes? Why or why not?
4. Discuss the issue of cost in connection with futile treatment.
5. How does quality of life fit in with this issue?
6. Should odds be a factor in determining whether or not treatment may be futile? Why or why not?
7. What was your reaction to the story about Melissa?
8. What was your reaction to the story about Kim?
9. What was your reaction to the story of Dr. L and Mr. M?
10. What are your views on the national trend concerning futile treatment?
11. What do you believe are the toughest types of cases involving futile treatment?
12. Discuss the difference between being in a coma and in a persistent vegetative state.

Activities / Group Discussion

1. List some factors to be considered in determining whether or not treatment may be futile.
2. Discuss under what circumstances a doctor should be able to override the wishes of next of kin.
3. Use newspapers or magazines to locate and discuss more cases of futile treatment.
4. What are the differences, if any, between a young child and elderly person concerning this issue?
5. Pro and con: All life is sacred and must be supported to the maximum.

PART 7: HEALTH CARE REFORM

Chapter Summary

- Elected officials face tough choices on health care rationing.
- When health care reform comes, it must correct our long-time neglect of those who can't care for themselves.
- Prices of medicine are rising faster than inflation.
- The high cost of medicine is a bioethics issue for many Americans.
- The topic of health care reform and rationing stirs up many emotions.

Discussion Questions

1. What new insights did you receive from reading this section?
2. In your own words, explain what health care reform means to you.
3. What is fair and unfair about health care rationing?
4. On what basis are rationing choices made? By whom?
5. What is your view of health care rationing?
6. What is the cause of the "doctor shuffle"?
7. What's most important to you in shopping for a physician?
8. In the article on poll watching, which poll outcomes were the most interesting?
9. What are polls saying about America's attitude toward health care reform?

10. How did you do on the health care pop quiz? What surprised you?
11. Give your reaction to the article on drug company costs and profits.
12. What is the most important health care reform issue for you? Why?

Activities / Group Discussion

1. Create a list of good and bad aspects of health care reform.
2. How would you reform health care? Create a list of reforms as a group.
3. Compare U.S. and Canadian health care.
4. You are 85 years old and in good health. What are your fears?
5. Your parent must go to a nursing home. List what needs to be done and considered.

PART 8: ISSUES IN MENTAL HEALTH

Chapter Summary

- Health care insurance does not cover most mental illnesses.
- As many as 80 percent of people with severe mental illness are treatable.
- Mental illness is made worse by stigma and guilt.
- Only a small percentage of mentally ill are dangerous to others.
- Mental illness afflicts 20 to 40 million Americans each year.

Discussion Questions

1. What new insights did you receive from reading this section?
2. What was your view of mental illness while growing up?
3. Why do you think mental illness is so misunderstood?
4. How has legislation helped and hindered the fight for mental health?
5. Why are insurance companies reluctant to pay for mental health coverage?
6. Why is there a shortage of halfway houses?
7. What are the costs of mental illness for a family? For society?

8. In your own words, explain the meaning of mental illness.
9. Why are we still blaming demons for mental illness?
10. How has mental illness touched your life?
11. What factors make mental illness hard to treat?
12. Why is it hard for politicians and the public to pay attention to mental illness?

Activities / Group Discussion

1. Create a list of mental health issues and prioritize them.
2. Research what kind of help is available in your area for mental illness.
3. List the different types of mental illness.
4. Discuss ways people can make a difference in improving mental health care.
5. Use local and national publications to locate articles on mental health issues.

PART 9: RESEARCH

Chapter Summary
- Americans have been unwittingly used as guinea pigs by scientists.
- Research experiments are sometimes falsely presented as therapy.
- Using humans for research is essential and we all owe something to it.
- Full knowledge of risk is essential to informed consent.
- "Defensive research" is often a loophole for biological weapons research.

Discussion Questions

1. What new insights did you receive from reading this section?
2. What issues are involved in voluntary consent?
3. Explain the appeal to scientists of the ethic "the greatest good for the greatest number."
4. In your own words, explain what "research" means to you.
5. Name some examples of unethical research.

6. What issues and concerns are raised by biological weapons?
7. How are ethics enforced in research?
8. Give some examples of unexpected consequences of research.
9. Give your reaction to fertility research and the issues it raises.
10. Explain how science is torn between the "big deal and big ideal."
11. What has been the history of use of biological weapons?
12. Explain the "defense research" loophole. How could this loophole be eliminated?

Activities / Group Discussion
1. Make a list of issues related to ethics in research.
2. Should doctors take part in medical research for the military? Explain.
3. Debate whether the U.S. should be involved in defensive research.
4. Discuss the thin line between justified and unjustified risks and research.
5. Brainstorm how citizens can get their voices heard concerning biological research issues.

PART 10: REFUSING TREATMENT

Chapter Summary
- Most doctors are aware of a patient's right to refuse treatment.
- The U.S. Supreme Court has ruled that a patient's right to refuse treatment is nearly absolute.
- The key question is often "what would the patient have wanted?"
- Technology drove the last nail into the coffin of doctor-dominated decision making.
- Our right to say no to death-prolonging technology has been getting stronger year by year.

Discussion Questions
1. What new insights did you receive from reading this section?
2. Give your reaction to the case regarding Hugh Finn.

3. Why were Barber and Nejdl charged with murder in the Herbert case?
4. What is the "mistaken legacy" of the Barber–Nejdl case?
5. Why don't most doctors today know the outcome of the Barber–Nejdl case?
6. What fiction sometimes prevents people from allowing someone to die?
7. What was the primary issue in the Karen Ann Quinlan case?
8. What issues are involved in the right to refuse treatment?
9. How can people protect their rights to refuse treatment?
10. For what reasons do some people want treatment continued no matter what?
11. What issues complicate the work of EMTs?
12. What was the result of *Barber versus the Supreme Court?*

Activities / Group Discussion

1. Discuss how patients could be better educated about refusing treatment.
2. Discuss how doctors could be better educated about a patient's right to refuse treatment.
3. How does the right to refuse treatment affect you?
4. How does the right to refuse treatment affect your family members?
5. Share your own personal feelings about this issue.

PART 11: ISSUES TO PONDER

Chapter Summary

- Cigarettes kill approximately 350,000 people per year.
- Smoking costs the U.S. health care system about $50 billion a year.
- National calamities raise questions about our response to human need.
- We are inconsistent about enforcing what protects us from ourselves.
- We regulate what we think we can enforce.

Discussion Questions

1. What new insights did you receive from reading this section?
2. How do you feel about the practice of selling human organs?
3. Under what circumstances would you sell a body part?
4. Under what circumstances would you buy a body part?
5. Under what circumstances would you donate an organ to help a family member or friend?
6. Why has it been illegal to sell organs?
7. What do you think about the 1999 Pennsylvania experiment?
8. Do you think bikers are being discriminated against by the requirement to wear helmets? Explain.
9. What prevents people from signing up as organ donors?
10. Why don't people get excited about long-term disasters? Give an example.
11. Give your reaction to the essay titled "Arithmetic Lesson."
12. Did you change your feelings about any of these issues as a result of this discussion?

Activities / Group Discussion

1. Discuss what is good and bad about the current organ donation system.
2. Debate: Do we discriminate against smokers by taxing cigarettes?
3. Debate: Why do we ban pot, but not booze?
4. Compile a list for and against banning cigarettes.
5. Discuss to what extent should the government limit our freedom in order to protect us from ourselves?

PART 12: VIOLENCE AS A HEALTH ISSUE

Chapter Summary
- We have a selective blindness about violence.
- Living free of violence is a fundamental right.
- Homicide is often the result of politics, emotion, and greed.
- People are often inconsistent by being pro-life on one issue and pro-death on another.

• Even when you are opposing a force that is morally wrong, you don't use morally questionable tactics.

Discussion Questions

1. What new insights did you receive from reading this section?
2. Why is violence a health issue? Explain.
3. Why can't we ignore violence? What happens when we do?
4. What types of violence do we often choose not to see?
5. In your own words, explain what "violence" means to you.
6. How have you been personally affected by violence?
7. What are some of the causes of spouse abuse?
8. Give your reaction to the essay "A Dubious Analogy."
9. What are your feelings about the competition between Edison and Westinghouse?
10. What does violence cost our society?
11. What do polls show about public support for the death penalty?
12. How are doctors sometimes involved in executions?

Activities / Group Discussion

1. Discuss how we are affected by violence on television.
2. Is there any difference in violence we see on the news as opposed to television shows and movies? Is any worse than the other?
3. Discuss issues raised by the death penalty.
4. Discuss effective ways to reduce violence.
5. What insights have you gained from reading this book and from these discussions?